2/15

The Infectious Microbe

The Infectious Microbe

William Firshein

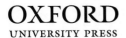

OXFORD
UNIVERSITY PRESS

OXFORD
UNIVERSITY PRESS

Oxford University Press is a department of the University of Oxford.
It furthers the University's objective of excellence in research, scholarship,
and education by publishing worldwide.

Oxford New York
Auckland Cape Town Dar es Salaam Hong Kong Karachi
Kuala Lumpur Madrid Melbourne Mexico City Nairobi
New Delhi Shanghai Taipei Toronto

With offices in
Argentina Austria Brazil Chile Czech Republic France Greece
Guatemala Hungary Italy Japan Poland Portugal Singapore
South Korea Switzerland Thailand Turkey Ukraine Vietnam

Oxford is a registered trade mark of Oxford University Press
in the UK and certain other countries.

Published in the United States of America by
Oxford University Press
198 Madison Avenue, New York, NY 10016

Library of Congress Cataloging-in-Publication Data
Firshein, William.
   The infectious microbe / William Firshein.
      p.   cm.
   Includes bibliographical references.
   ISBN 978–0–19–932961–8 (alk. paper)
   I. Title.
   [DNLM: 1. Microbiological Phenomena. 2. Bioterrorism—prevention & control.
3. Communicable Diseases, Emerging. 4. Microbiology—history. 5. Virulence Factors. QW 4]
   QR46
   616.9'041—dc23
                                                          2013017114
9780199329618

29.95

9 8 7 6 5 4 3 2 1

Printed in the United States of America on acid-free paper

CONTENTS

PREFACE

Of the almost innumerable interactions between science and humanity, few are as central as the life sciences, and in particular, the microbial world. This world is immense and includes a tremendous variety of microscopic creatures, such as bacteria, fungi, actinomycetes (organisms that lie midway between bacteria and fungi), viruses, and protozoa, among many other groups. Because they are so intimately involved with life on this planet, they must be taken into account in many ways when considering the public good. Such concerns include their historical role in infectious diseases (e.g., bubonic plague in the Middle Ages and the Spanish influenza pandemic after World War I), as well as their roles in pollution; cycles of nature; climate change; bioterrorism; fermentation (e.g., production of alcohol from yeast and antibiotics by other microorganisms); industrial microbiology; food spoilage (e.g., botulism poisoning in incompletely sterilized canned foods); animal, plant, and crop health; soil fertility; exploration of new oil deposits; genetic engineering (e.g., production of vital hormones such as insulin); space exploration; origin of life; and yes, even normal development of healthy human beings and animals. Just as a few vivid examples: 1) If microorganisms did not exist, every living organism that ever died would still be here. They would not decay, and life could not sustain itself. Only because of the incredible metabolic activities of certain groups of microorganisms do the cells and tissues of dead organisms "break down" chemically and return to their basic molecular forms to be used by other living organisms for their own growth and development. 2) There is no naturally occurring sterile environment that exists for living organisms on this planet. All living beings are in intimate association with myriads of microorganisms that change with time both in types and numbers. However, artificial germ-free environments can be constructed for research and medical purposes. One purpose involves analyzing what happens to animals born into such an artificial environment. The result is ultimately fatal for them because their immune (defense) capabilities (against infectious diseases) and digestive systems do not develop normally. They require appropriate microorganisms to activate both metabolic systems accurately (a result of evolution).

Even if one was not aware of all the activities of microorganisms described above, and even if it was unclear why the activities of the vast majority of microorganisms are beneficial and absolutely essential for our existence, it is almost certain that their harmful capabilities in causing serious and sometimes fatal diseases are well known and feared. From diseases caused by bacteria, such as pneumonia, tuberculosis, anthrax, scarlet fever, tetanus, meningitis, typhoid, cholera, dysentery, and bubonic plague (among many others), to diseases caused by viruses, such as HIV (AIDS), polio, yellow fever, colds, hepatitis, rabies, and influenza (flu) (among many others), humanity has struggled to cope with their ever-changing capabilities. That is because the evolution of microorganisms is a billion-fold faster than our own evolution, which results constantly in emerging diseases that we have never faced before. Thus, our defense (immune) capabilities have had to evolve also to "combat" these new "aggressors." Fortunately, technology has enabled us to develop aids to our own defense systems, such as antibiotics. Nevertheless, such abuses as the indiscriminate overuse of these "wonder drugs" have reached an alarming state of futility, since the pathogens (disease-producing microorganisms) have become resistant to their killing effects by the process of mutation and selection or by other genetic mechanisms.

This book has been written in order to help readers understand all the scientific concepts and terminology of how microbial or viral diseases are caused, or to intelligently ask questions about or discuss the impact of such diseases on our well-being, or to comprehend reports about disease outbreaks in the news media, which appear daily. I believe this work, in the form of a narrative, is unique because both life science majors and nonmajors, as well as specialized other constituencies, such as nurses or life science majors in community college, can benefit from its content. How is this broad spectrum possible? First, the text is based on courses that I have taught to majors and nonmajors in mixed and separate venues for more than fifty years at Wesleyan University. Thus, I have mixed what I consider the perfect cocktail of scientific detail and broad concepts that are required for both constituencies to absorb. The nonscientist will not be put off by the "hard" science (which includes a basic understanding of molecular genetics, molecular biology, and biochemistry) because the prose is, I hope, clear, enthusiastic, and concise—a style I've relied on during my life as a teacher and researcher, and there are many colored images to help the student relate to the discussion. Moreover, there are numerous connections to the broader picture of infectiousness. The science major should also appreciate the scientific concepts and details, which are not much different than those found in much-larger microbiology texts in the major. I have simply distilled them down to their bare essentials, while also including an extensive glossary of definitions. As for the other specialized constituencies, community college students and nurses, all could benefit from this work in different ways: the former as described above, and the latter as an introduction to infectious diseases and what a nurse should know about pathogens.

The heart of the book describes in great detail the pathogenicity of six very important diverse microbes, for two reasons. One, I wished to show that all these pathogens follow the basic dogma, if you will, of infectiousness: namely, invasion, internal spread, toxin effects, and excretion (spread). Two, it is unnecessary, therefore, to describe in detail the plethora of other microbes to gain a basic understanding of pathogenicity. Other aspects in the book include a brief but essential historical review to understand how far we have come, and how far we yet have to go to elucidate and appreciate the scope of pathogenicity; a basic overview of genetics (including molecular genetics), molecular biology, and biochemistry, as well as how microbes metabolize and "grow"; a discussion of a relatively new concept in the way microbes exist as a community in nature and in many disease states (biofilms); the concepts of emerging and reemerging diseases; and as an extra bonus, the myths and realities of bioterrorism, one of the powerful offshoots of infection.

William Firshein
Department of Molecular Biology and Biochemistry
Wesleyan University

ACKNOWLEDGMENTS

I am grateful beyond measure for the help of Debby Alexson, who spent much of her valuable free time typing my manuscript, retyping it after I inserted corrections, and getting it in shape for transmission to the appropriate literary venues. Without her invaluable aid, I never would have realized my dream.

A number of others acted as advisors for this work, none more so than my colleague Don Oliver, who suggested that I put my teaching expertise of fifty years at Wesleyan University into this type of endeavor in order to open up the important world of microbiology to nonmajors, the public, and other specialized groups such as nurses and students in community colleges. Of course, nothing that I wrote would have meant anything without the important assistance of the Jennifer Lyons Literary Agency, and Jeff Ourvan of this agency, who worked earnestly to present my work to a large number of qualified publishers in the best possible light. I also want to praise Jennifer Lyons for her confidence in my approach to the book and for choosing Oxford University Press as a possible publisher, which was a stroke of great insight on Jennifer's part. Such insight enabled me to come under the excellent care of Jeremy Lewis, the copyeditor at Oxford, and Erik Hane, the assistant copyeditor, both of whom helped me in many ways to complete all that was required for the book to be published, with the able assistance of Karen Jessie the project manager from Integra one of the partner production companies of Oxford. Grateful appreciation goes to John Wareham, who prepared some of the photographs and other artwork, and to Millie Marmur, who provided me with help in searching out the best agency. I am grateful to the Wasch Center for Retired Faculty at Wesleyan University and to its director, Karl Scheibe, who offered me a "home" and a quiet corner to complete my book. I thank my long-time great friend Paul Schwaber for being my "friend" and always encouraging me to fight the good fight against adversity. Other colleagues in the Departments of Biology and Molecular Biology and Biochemistry (here or passed on), including Anthony (Tony) Infante, Lew Lukens, Jason Wolfe, Barry Kiefer, and Spencer Berry, provided an atmosphere of good will and friendship that enabled me to prosper in my professional discipline of microbiology and aided me immensely in becoming a better colleague.

Last, but certainly not least, is my wife, Anna. You are the best. I have been blessed in so many ways with our children, but none more so than being together with you for so many wonderful years. You have provided me with the care, affection, and happiness that enabled me to forge ahead when difficulties sprang up. I could not have accomplished anything without you at my side.

The Infectious Microbe

1

Introduction to the Infectious Microbe

A. The Scope of Microbial Life and Infectious Diseases

There is no real estimate or knowledge of how many microorganisms exist in our world. In a way, an exploration of the universe of bacteria, fungi, yeasts, and other microbes is, as Captain Kirk used to say on *Star Trek*, "the final frontier," but it is a frontier in a largely unknown universe of microorganisms that inhabit every nook and cranny of our own microcosm of a world, from the deepest trenches in the oceans to the outer reaches of our atmosphere, including the North and South Poles. Even in inhospitable environments such as those boiling (100 degrees centigrade) pools in Yellowstone National Park, to the Dead Sea in Israel (which has a concentration of salt that reaches saturation of 29%), and to sulfur mines where sulfuric acid is present in high concentrations, microbiologists can isolate microorganisms that thrive. That is a remarkable observation in itself. It becomes even more remarkable when one includes estimates of actual numbers of such microorganisms. Because these living creatures are microscopic (and make no mistake about it, they are living, complete organisms but consist of only one cell, the fundamental unit of life), there can be uncounted numbers even in one gram of soil. However, in an analysis that was recently made in one ton of soil, the staggering total exceeded by 100,000 times the number of stars in our galaxy (ten to the sixteenth power bacteria, that is, sixteen zeros after the numeral one, compared to ten to the eleventh power for the number of stars). Figures 1.1–1.3 depict examples of some common bacteria, showing their extremely small size (Figure 1.2) and where they exist (Figures 1.1, 1.3).

Such numbers are hard to contemplate, and they are staggering when one realizes that is in only *one ton* of soil. Of course, there are other environments closer to "home," such as our own bodies, where equally as staggering numbers can be found. Thus, the gastrointestinal tract alone of a normal adult human

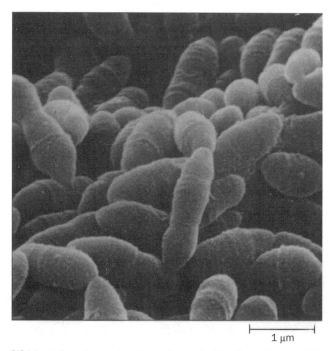

FIGURE 1.1 *Bifidobacterium*, the dominant bacterium in the intestines of breastfed infants.

being contains over four hundred different species of bacteria, and their "weight" (an indirect measure of numbers) would be about one kilogram (one thousand grams, or 2.2 pounds) of bacteria. That computes to more "foreign" living cells in the form of microorganisms than there are cells that make up

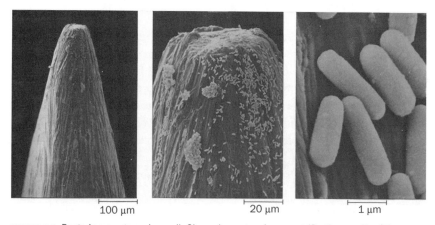

FIGURE 1.2 Bacteria are extremely small. Shown here at various magnifications, cells of the bacterium *Bacillus subtilis* on the tip of a pin. In the scale, μm is a "micrometer" (one millionth of a meter, which is 39.37 inches). (See Plate 1)

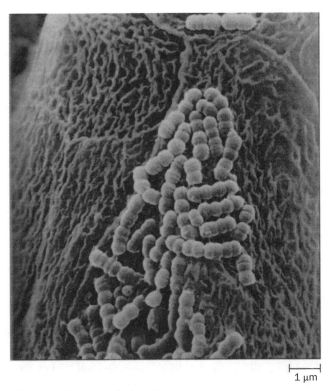

1 μm

FIGURE 1.3 Adherence of bacteria to body surfaces.

our own bodies. The important concept that emerges from these "statistical" facts is that every living multicellular organism (that includes "us" as well as other mammals, birds, fish, reptiles, plants, insects, sponges, ferns, and many other organisms) is in intimate association with myriads of microorganisms. There is no naturally occurring sterile environment that we can move around without being in contact with them. Interestingly enough, however, germ-free environments can be constructed for research and medical purposes. One such purpose involves analyzing what happens to animals that are born into an artificial situation. This type of birth procedure is not good at all, since their immune capabilities and digestive systems do not develop normally—we need them to survive! A second purpose is for medical reasons, to help sustain those poor individuals who have genetic or other defects in their immune systems. Any exposure to the normal world would "contaminate" the victims with microorganisms and would overwhelm their immune capabilities. An example was the boy living in a plastic germ-free bubble, which was the subject of a TV movie some time ago. From many studies such as those above, a new concept of the "microbiome" has arisen, remarkably, that microbes in our body, primarily in the gastrointestinal tract but in other places as well, such as the mouth and nasopharynx, "cooperate" with our much-larger cells to maintain our health. This concept goes on to assert that human or animal cells are just one (albeit important) member of this immense community. Thus, besides helping the digestive system and immune system to develop normally, as described above, these microbes are vital in other ways as well, such as synthesizing vitamins (in the digestive tract) that our own cells cannot make, and destroying alien microbes capable of causing disease. They just wipe them out by secreting their own lethal factors. Now that's cooperation! Their importance is further emphasized by the fact that if the microbiome is depleted of "beneficial microbes," such as by the overuse of antibiotics, then other maladies can result, such as obesity, heart disease, asthma, and gastrointestinal upsets. Another important concept that underlies our association with microorganisms is that it is not a static phenomenon. The same numbers and types of microorganisms do not exist for any length of time in our bodies. They are constantly changing both in types and numbers. Our relationships with these amazing organisms are also forever evolving, which means that not only do we have to adapt to them, but they to us as well. Now that is a "mutual" relationship. Nevertheless, the much more numerous microorganisms are evolving much faster than we are because they multiply (divide) so quickly and can reach astounding numbers in a very short time, producing many variants or new types (mutants) not present previously. From even one live bacterial cell, after twenty-four hours as many as fifty million can be present in a small culture volume. In fact, it has been calculated that the pace of microbial evolution is one billion times greater than that of human beings. Fortunately, most of these microbial types (species) will never be in contact with us, but because of our modern industrial society, we are coming into contact with more and more of them. That is, we are being exposed to new environments and new physical and atmospheric conditions such as pollution and global warming that could put us on a collision course with new and unusual microorganisms, with which we may or may not interact. Nevertheless, it is worth keeping in mind that the human species has existed in its current form for over 200,000 years (give or take a few tens of thousands of years), and we have survived this incredible onslaught of microorganisms up until now.

B. What Is a Pathogen?

The sixty-four-thousand-dollar question (we used to call it the sixty-four-dollar question when I was growing up) is why should we be worried about interacting with microorganisms? I did point out above that many of them intimately associated with us are essential for normal development of our immune systems and even our digestion. Unfortunately, I am certain that even if you never even knew what a microorganism was before or never participated in any science course in which microorganisms were discussed, you were probably aware that some of them can cause serious and sometimes fatal diseases. These include pneumonia, meningitis, scarlet fever, tuberculosis, AIDS, influenza (flu), rabies, smallpox, polio, yellow fever, typhus, typhoid, cholera, leprosy, bubonic plague, anthrax, tetanus, botulism, and many more. And this is only a very small sample. In fact, until I cited some good characteristics of microorganisms, you probably had the impression only that they were "bad" because they caused infectious diseases. They made us "sick." Well, you should not be "criticized" for your impression, although we know now that there are many more beneficial activities such as cycles of nature, soil fertility, fermentation, and decay in which microorganisms are involved that are essential for the survival of all living creatures on this planet. Throughout history, microbial interactions with humans were almost always viewed as negative. The golden age of microbiology began in the nineteenth century, when it was discovered that specific diseases were caused by specific microorganisms. Many historical accounts have been written describing the terrible plague (bubonic) in the Middle Ages, which wiped out a quarter of the population in Europe, or the flu pandemic after World War I, which killed over twenty million people. Most wars up until World War II resulted in more casualties from bacterial or bacterial-like and viral infections than from combat. World War I was particularly devastating because there were no real antibacterial drugs to treat deep wounds. The French general Napoleon lost most of his great army to diseases such as typhus when he invaded Russia and then had to retreat from Moscow, the capital. Thus, as has been written in several famous books, such as *Rats, Lice and History* by Hans Zinsser, the *Microbe Hunters* by Paul DeKruif, and *Guns, Germs, and Steel* by Jared Diamond, it would be safe to say that microbial diseases helped shape our own human history dramatically, at the same time reinforcing our negative "opinion" of microorganisms. Even today, microbe-human interactions are accentuated in a distinctly negative manner by advertising "anti-bacterial" or even "anti-viral" consumer products, from mouthwashes to kitchen cleaners.

C. The Relationship between a Pathogen and the Host It Infects Is Complex and Varied

Although there is a strong belief by most of us that microbial diseases are always dangerous and are a one-way street toward sickness or death, that is many times not the case. Rather, a microbial "disease" is best characterized as a "relationship" between the microorganism (called a pathogen; that is, a microorganism capable of causing a disease) and the host (the individual with whom it comes in contact, or infects). Because the term "pathogen" implies a successful outcome for the microorganism, which isn't always the case, a microbial infection is more aptly described as a "host-parasite" relationship, where "parasite" is defined as any organism that is sheltered or feeds in a different organism. It does not necessarily imply that the infection will always lead to a successful outcome for the parasite. In fact, there are three outcomes of an infection by a microorganism: (1) the parasite becomes a pathogen and overcomes the immune defenses of the host, (2) the host's immune defenses overcome the ability of the potential pathogen to cause the disease, or (3) most intriguing, the parasite (or potential pathogen) and the host survive together (why in the world would they want to do that?). These are the three extremes for this relationship, and they depend on many, many diverse factors. For example, potential pathogens fall into two basic types, primary and opportunistic. The former can often cause diseases among a definite percentage of infected individuals, while the latter causes diseases only in individuals whose immune systems are temporarily or permanently defective. Nevertheless, an opportunistic pathogen in one host can be a primary one in another. What makes a pathogen successful? Basically, it is a combination of its own "prowess"; that is, an ability to produce virulence (or poisonous) factors that damage the host, and the "weakness" of the host's immune defenses. In some cases the immune defense system is strong, but the virulence factors produced by the pathogen are still more powerful. Nevertheless, it is not always the case that success will result in the demise of the host. In most cases, the host becomes sick but eventually rallies to overcome the virulence of the pathogen, resulting in its destruction, although in many cases, the pathogen can exist in low numbers in various parts of the body. Even if the host's immune system is compromised this outcome can occur, but it will take longer. It is like a race, one that pits the specific response of the immune system to the pathogen (which takes time to develop) against the growth and multiplication of the pathogen (which also takes time). However, it is the third outcome, where a relationship is established between the host and the parasite, that has led to new thinking about pathogenicity. In one sense, it does not make evolutionary "sense" for the potential pathogen to "destroy" its host, because without a suitable host, the pathogen too will become extinct. Thus, in the long run, pathogens have an "interest" in ensuring the host's survival. As a famous Nobel Prize microbiologist, Joshua Lederberg, has written, "We should think of each host and its parasite as a super organism" where "domesticating the host is the better long term strategy for the parasite" (imagine humans being "domesticated" by microorganisms!). Thus, many diseases have evolved into "milder" sicknesses, such as *Streptococcus pyogenes*. (Names or nomenclature of specific microorganisms are derived from a binomial-component system used commonly in the biological sciences, with two epithets: "genus" and "species." Thus, *Streptococcus* denotes the genus; *pyogenes*, the species.) This particular microorganism causes, among other ailments, the common "strep" sore throat. Yet, during the twentieth century, infections that started with this symptom progressed many times to scarlet fever, which could be fatal, and further to rheumatic fever, a debilitating chronic disease that could permanently damage the heart. In a strange twist of fate, in 1901 the famous Rockefeller Institute for Medical Research was founded by John D. Rockefeller because his grandson died of scarlet fever and he was determined to find ways to treat this and other diseases such as pneumonia, for which there were no cures. Today, although these diseases still exist, they are, except for the "strep" throat, exceedingly rare because of the genetic alteration in the ability of this streptococcus to produce one or more virulence factors. Nevertheless, such changes would probably have not led to the survival of the less dangerous microorganism unless it was advantageous, as, for example, not destroying its host. Of interest is that such changes may also occur within a relatively short time period. A striking example could involve one of the most dreaded diseases of our time, caused by the HIV virus (or human immunodeficiency virus), which eventually leads to AIDS (or acquired immunodeficiency syndrome). Although the results are by necessity preliminary, it appears that HIV caused a more rapid progression to full-blown AIDS during the late 1970s and 1980s than it does now (2000–present). Newer samples of the virus do not develop well in the host cells (lymphocytes, which are white blood cells) they infect and are not as resistant to immune attack as those preserved from patients in those previous years. Thus, passage of the virus in the general human population has possibly made it "weaker" with time, perhaps reaching an "equilibrium" with its host to "permit" a longer survival period. This, of course, is not meant to imply that the "virus" has some kind of purposeful thought process; rather, it suggests some kind of natural process that has evolved with time that affects both the host and the parasite. This process is called "natural selection." Indeed, there are numerous examples of a host modification that can render it more resistant to a particular pathogen, even if the modification results in a genetic defect. One such classic example involves the parasite that causes malaria (a protozoan—still a microorganism). It has great difficulty infecting those individuals who have sickle cell anemia (in which red blood cells are deformed), because as part of its life cycle, the parasite must grow in normal red blood cells. Another example concerns the virus we mentioned above— HIV. In order to infect susceptible lymphocytes, it must first attach to certain "receptor" sites on the surface of the lymphocyte. In the alteration, which is not known to be harmful to the host, the components that make up the receptor sites have been changed by some type of genetic event (mutation?) during evolution of some of our ancestors, which prevents the virus from binding. Thus, this subset of our population is immune to the development of AIDS or at least is more resistant to the development of AIDS.

Nevertheless, not all is "perfect" in this model of mutual benefits for host and parasite. There are many exceptions, among which is the phenomenon of "zoonoses," which involves the transfer of the parasite from its natural host to a new species. In many, but not all, of these transfers, the accidental new host is primarily a "dead end" where no further direct transmission can occur. Some well-known examples for humans include rabies, which is caused by a virus transmitted from a bite (usually by an infected animal or bat); inhalation anthrax, which is a disease of wild and domestic animals that is caused by a bacterium, *Bacillus anthracis*, that is spread through the air by spores and deposited eventually into the lungs; and Lyme disease, which is caused by a bacterium called a spirochete that is spread by the bite of a tick that had previously infected mice or deer. A striking example of zoonoses in which further spread can occur in the accidental host is AIDS.

D. Susceptibility and Virulence Factors Are Closely Related

In our previous discussion, we spoke of the "prowess" of a potential pathogen to cause disease; namely, an ability to produce virulence (or poisonous) factors that overcome host defenses. However, not all the virulence factors are "poisonous" per se, but rather they act to ensure that the potential pathogen can successfully invade the organs or tissues of its host, where it can exert its poisonous effects. In fact, there is a defined sequence of steps that almost all pathogens must follow to ensure this outcome (with a few more steps thrown in to ensure its spread and maintenance). These include an ability (1) to invade or enter a host, (2) to establish itself in a specific niche (site) in the host, (3) to avoid or subvert host immune defenses, or cause them to act abnormally, (4) to multiply extensively at its primary niche or spread to secondary sites and multiply, (5) to produce and deliver toxins into host cells (the actual component or components that are poisonous to the host), and (6) to be transmitted to a new host, or to be maintained in the host it has infected even after the host has been cured. As a famous specialist in microbial diseases, Stanley Falkow, put it, pathogenicity "can be likened to a symphony in which each part contributes to a common theme." There are several important ramifications of this list. First is that despite the existence of many different types of pathogens, most seem to be subject to this common strategy for causing the disease. Second, the many virulence factors that have been detected thus far seem mostly to share similar mechanisms of action or properties, despite the fact that their chemical compositions and structures may be different. Third, an understanding of how these virulence factors act can lead to the design or development of a general or universal method of treating diverse infectious diseases.

Before we delve into the nature of these virulence factors in more detail, to gain a better understanding of their activities, an important concept to discuss is that of host "susceptibility," a term that is vital to understanding whether the virulence factors will be able to be made in sufficient amounts and/or to function. Usually, most human beings are healthy. Some imbalance to the feeling of health must occur to a host, transiently or permanently, to tip the balance for or against a successful microbial disease. Many of the causes for this imbalance are vague and poorly understood, but ultimately they must come down most probably to a malfunction of the immune defenses that control the infection, and the special properties of the pathogen itself. The common adages "I feel run down and tired" or "I feel stressed out" are typical oversimplified statements that can result in becoming more susceptible to an infection. Such feelings may be traceable to a temporary lowering of immune defenses. There are, of course, many other factors for which we have little explanation that relate, for example, to the environment (such as colds in the winter, polio in the summer), or to predisposing genetic factors such as asthma that enable pathogens to overcome a weakened individual.

Returning to our description of virulence factors, the first two involve factors necessary for pathogens to invade and establish themselves in the host, or if they are already present in low numbers at various sites such as the nasopharynx (nose and throat), to migrate to the site of their primary infection (such as the lungs for the organism that causes pneumonia, *Streptococcus pneumoniae*). The list is not exhaustive, but in general they involve substances known as "adhesins," which help the pathogen to attach like a glue to sites on the surface of the host cells—not only the ultimate cells they intend to infect, but cells where they first come into contact with the host, either new or as long-term residents (again using the pneumonia example, cells of the nasopharynx initially, and cells in the lung eventually). Such adhesins are usually found at the tip of fibers that extend out from the surface of the bacterial cell; they are called "fimbrae" or "pili." Many times, however, the pathogen also must be able to degrade (break down or break through) barriers, such as connective tissue between cells that prevents it from reaching its internal target. These components are known generally as "invasins" and consist of special proteins called enzymes, which bind to a specific component known as a "substrate" and either degrade it (break it down into smaller components) or modify it to produce an end product that is different from the substrate. In the case of invasins, the substrate is a specific part of the barrier complex. Three such invasin enzymes include "hyaluronidase," which degrades connective tissues, "lecithinase," which degrades fats or lipids in a barrier, and "collagenase," which degrades the main component of bone collagen.

The next group of virulence factors encompasses a wide variety of mechanisms that the pathogen uses for "general survival." They differ depending on the pathogen, the site of infection, the specific host, and host immune defenses. Starting with the latter, many pathogens produce components that enable them to resist phagocytosis (engulfment by specific types of white blood cells that destroy the pathogen afterward). In effect, they coat themselves with a capsule that prevents or inhibits phagocytosis. Most capsules are composed of different types of polysaccharides, which are sugars linked together in a large polymer or proteins that are synthesized by the pathogen and secreted outside the cell. Another mechanism pathogens use to resist host defenses occurs by a phenomenon known as "phase variation." Many of them are capable through genetic means of altering their surface components, which are the primary sites by which the "workers" of the immune system (known as antibodies, proteins produced by specific white blood cells called plasma cells that circulate in the blood) are able to recognize that the pathogen is "foreign." The antibodies then bind strongly to these surface sites so that the pathogen can be sensitized for further processing and ultimate destruction. However, if the surface sites are altered, the antibodies that have been generated by the immune system to recognize the original surface components cannot do so and must be generated all over again, which takes time, allowing the pathogen to establish itself. There are also numerous survival mechanisms that involve nutrition, which enables the pathogen to multiply. This capability is among the most important of the virulence factors that we mentioned previously, because the pathogens must reach sufficient numbers in the host to produce the factors they need, such as the adhesins, invasins, capsules, etc. In other words, because pathogens are "cells" they require all the nutrients (vitamins, amino acids, sugars, and minerals) that our own cells need as well. How do they compete or "sequester" (concentrate) such nutrients for their own purposes? One example is that of iron, an important mineral required by all cells for energy metabolism. Yet, iron is very toxic when floating around free in the body. It must be complexed or hidden by our cells to prevent it from exerting its toxic action (hemoglobin in red blood cells is an example of complexed iron). Pathogens accomplish this feat by producing their own complex called a siderophore, which can compete much more efficiently for the iron that is present in complexes made by host cells or for the scarce free iron that may also be present. These bacterial "siderophores" bind iron tightly and then incorporate them into their own cells. Of course, there are also many nutrients that are floating around the body, which the pathogen can simply incorporate into its own cells, such as vitamins, amino acids, and purines and pyrimidines (building blocks for the nucleic acids DNA and RNA). Nutrients can also be derived in greater amounts from the destruction of cells and tissues by toxins, which releases them into the circulatory system and other sites. To augment such levels even further, many pathogens can form (or synthesize) these precursors themselves, using their own metabolic capabilities. Nevertheless, a number of them are defective in such synthesis. It is amazing, however, that such defects can be overcome if the specific precursor is one of the nutrients already present in the internal environment. Under these conditions the defective pathogen, which is termed an auxotroph because the defect is caused by a genetic mutation, can simply incorporate the specific component into its own cells for further processing. A classic example of pathogenic auxotrophy is that of some types of typhoid, caused by *Salmonella typhimurium*, which require preformed purines in order to cause the disease.

Now, we come to the "pièce de résistance" (as it is called), the production of toxins that cause and perpetuate most of the damage to the host. I say "most" because it has become very clear that for many pathogens, additional damage results from the host's own inflammatory response to the pathogen, which is defined as secretion of cellular factors known as "cytokines." These components can destroy many different kinds of cells and tissues as well. Toxin formation presents a dilemma for the pathogen—if too-much toxin is produced (and this can occur as greater numbers of cells are produced during multiplication, resulting in too much damage), the host can succumb. Thus, a delicate balance has to be worked out, where the production of toxin(s) is modulated so that the niche provided by the host for the pathogen remains intact. This situation does not occur all the time, such as with dead-end diseases such as rabies, but is sufficiently documented to represent an important outcome of the disease. Thus, there are many metabolic signaling devices that have evolved to shut down or decrease the amount of toxin(s) produced when enough toxin has been synthesized, resulting in a feedback loop of suppression. One of these loops involves the requirement for scarce iron (as we discussed previously), where toxin formation kills host cells that release iron, which is then sequestered by the pathogen's siderophore. When sufficient siderophores are formed, free iron decreases, and this decrease serves as a signal to cease toxin formation. What are toxins made of? A great majority are proteins, also enzymes that destroy host cells at extremely low concentration. In a number of cases, toxin formation can serve several purposes, including damage to the host and dispersal of the pathogens into the environment, enabling them to infect new hosts as well as providing a rich source of nutrients by destroying cells and tissues (as stated above). A classic example is cholera, caused by *Vibrio cholerae*, which induces a severe watery diarrhea causing the "excretion" of many liters of fluids containing the organism. There are basically two types of toxins, called exotoxins and endotoxins. The first is characterized by secretion of the toxin outside the cell, which can be disseminated by diffusion to reach the host cell or can be injected by a remarkable syringe-like structure created by the pathogen for this purpose, right into the host cell directly. Figures 1.4 and 1.5 depict how different types of exotoxins act, either to penetrate the host cell (Figure 1.4) or to damage the ability of the immune system to work properly (Figure 1.5).

The second type is actually part of the surface of the pathogenic cell itself but, interestingly enough, is also produced by nonpathogenic bacteria. It is composed of lipids (fats) and polysaccharides (linked sugar molecules) that protrude from the outermost part of the bacterial cells. Such endotoxins are usually not as toxic as exotoxins and depend on large numbers of cells to exert their damaging effects. Also of importance is that endotoxins have

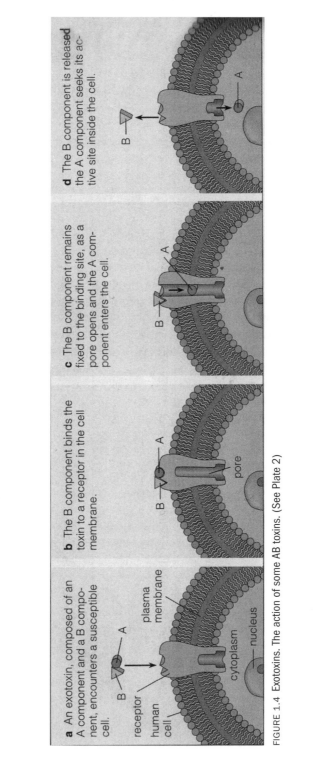

a An exotoxin, composed of an A component and a B component, encounters a susceptible cell.

B — ◢
A — ●

plasma membrane
receptor
human cell

cytoplasm
nucleus

b The B component binds the toxin to a receptor in the cell membrane.

B — ◢
A — ●

pore

c The B component remains fixed to the binding site, as a pore opens and the A component enters the cell.

B — ◢
A

d The B component is released the A component seeks its active site inside the cell.

B — ◢
A — ●

FIGURE 1.4 Exotoxins. The action of some AB toxins. (See Plate 2)

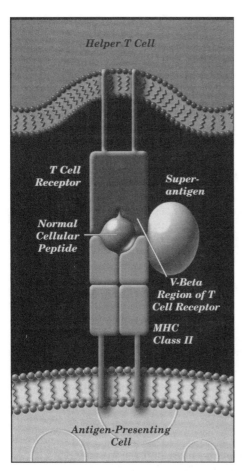

Helper T Cell

T Cell
Receptor

Super-
antigen

Normal
Cellular
Peptide

V-Beta
Region of T
Cell Receptor

MHC
Class II

Antigen-Presenting
Cell

FIGURE 1.5 Superantigens. These exotoxins act to short circuit the specificity of those white blood cells (known as helper "T" lymphocytes and macrophages) that bring the foreign substance (in this case, a fragment of the invading pathogen, known as the antigen) to the attachment site of the "T" lymphocyte, causing them to overproduce inflammatory factors that can damage or destroy host cells. (See Plate 3)

other properties besides their toxicity, such as inducing a significant increase in all kinds of immune reactions, which may have some positive applications in immunosuppressed individuals. However, getting back to exotoxins, some of them are among the most potent toxins ever produced by living cells, such as the toxin produced by the organism that causes botulism (*Clostridium botulinum*). It has been calculated that half a gram of pure toxin, if subdivided into six–billion-plus doses (the entire world's population), would kill all of us. Sadly, this toxin has been listed as a prime bioterror weapon. Other exotoxins secreted by pathogens that cause diphtheria (*Corynebacterium diphtheriae*), tetanus (*Clostridium tetani*), and cholera display most of the clinical properties of the disease. Also important to recognize is that many pathogens produce more, much more, than one kind of toxin—sometimes up to ten, such as the pathogen that causes bubonic plague (*Yersinia pestis*). Exotoxins can be classified in many ways, such as by what host cells or what part of the host cell they affect. These include neurotoxins, which affect nerve cells, membrane-damaging toxins, which disrupt the special structure that controls permeability of host cells, toxins that damage immune cells called superantigens (Figure 1.5), and a number of other specialized exotoxins. Many but not all exotoxins are known as "A-B" toxins, in that they consist of two parts: the active or toxic part (A) and the other, "nontoxic" part (B), which is essential for binding to specific receptors on the host cell to enable the toxic A subunit to enter the targeted cell (Figure 1.4). As you can sense, there are many aspects of toxin formation and activity, which we can only broach, but our discussion has highlighted many of them.

Finally, the last of the virulence factors stated in a previous section concerns how the pathogen is disseminated. One mechanism, that of cholera, was described above, but there are many other diverse routes that pathogens use to leave their host and to infect a new one. For most of the pathogens that cause respiratory infections such as pneumonia, influenza, colds, and tuberculosis, they are released by "violent" acts, such as sneezing or coughing or simply by breathing. For gastrointestinal infections, the route of dissemination is through the bowels. Other routes of dissemination involve unsafe sexual practices or drug use with contaminated needles. These include HIV (AIDS), syphilis, gonorrhea, and genital herpes. Then there are other specialized routes of dissemination that involve insect vectors (mosquitoes in particular) to spread diseases such as malaria, yellow fever, West Nile disease, and bubonic plague (fleas). Additional discussion of all these virulence factors will occur in the special topics of specific diseases.

E. Major Groups of Pathogens Are Found throughout the Microbial World

In our previous discussions concerning pathogenicity, we have not distinguished among different major groups of pathogens, using examples that cut across the entire range of microorganisms, especially viruses, which some microbiologists call nonliving infectious agents. Although an extensive discussion of all these groups lies outside the scope and purpose of this book, it is important to at least briefly describe those that harbor pathogens. A simplistic but effective way in which we categorize them is whether they are "free living" (that is, capable of being cultivated outside their hosts in artificial nutrient solutions, which we call "in vitro") or can be cultured only inside living cells (which we call "in vivo"). Within bacteria, although most pathogens can be cultured in vitro, some produce their deadly toxins only by growing in vivo, while others are not capable of being cultured in vitro, but only in vivo. Pathogens that cause typhoid, dysentery, and other gastrointestinal diseases represent examples of the former, while typhus and Rocky Mountain spotted fever represent examples of the latter. The causative agents of these latter diseases are small bacteria called rickettsia, which are carried by ticks and lice that transmit them by biting their human prey. As stated previously, more casualties in wars (up until the First World War [1914–1918]) were probably caused by typhus than by actual combat. However, there is an inspiring saga connected with the discovery of these two diseases as well; namely, the self sacrifice of two early microbiologists, Howard Ricketts (for whom the genus is named) and Stanislaus Prowazek (for whom the species that causes typhus, *Rickettsia prowazekii*, is named). In studying typhus during the early 1900s, both of them contracted it and died almost at the same time and at the same early age, thirty-nine. Now, these diseases can be successfully treated with antibiotics, although, sadly, they were not available then.

There are two other large groups of microorganisms whose pathogenic members are capable of being cultured in vitro that lie outside the "kingdom" of bacteria; namely, actinomycetes and fungi (although some microbiologists consider the former to be bacterial in origin). Fungi are made up of a huge heterogeneous and variable group of "micro" organisms, including mushrooms, which are not microscopic, and yeast, which provides humanity with wonderful "nutritional" benefits such as cheese and wine due to their ability to ferment (chemically decompose) various sugars. Their main form of growth (except for yeast) occurs via extensive branched filaments, usually in the soil. Strictly speaking, they do not consist of "one" cell like a bacterium but are usually made of long chains of millions of cells that contain structures such as nuclei (where the chromosomes with their DNA are contained), which do not exist in true bacteria. At various sites along the filaments, fruiting bodies develop that produce spores. Only yeasts exist as single cells with nuclei (and spores). A large number of fungi cause diseases of plants, while only a few cause major diseases in animals and humans. Unfortunately, when the immune system is compromised in a sick individual, it is then that fungal diseases become most dangerous, because their spores can be ingested through the nose or mouth and germinate (begin to grow) in vulnerable individuals. Fungi can cause diseases in several ways, such as (1) by inducing an allergic reaction to fungal spores (such as hay fever and asthma), (2) by actually growing on the skin (such as athlete's foot), and (3) by producing toxins such as ergot, which has been known since the Middle Ages and is probably the basis for the "witches of Salem" bewitchment of teenagers suffering from convulsions in the late 1600s, which resulted in the burning of helpless women accused of witchcraft. However, other fungal toxins cause severe diseases such as histoplasmosis (which resembles tuberculosis because of the growth of the fungi in the lungs), brain meningitis (an almost 100% fatal infection of the lining of the brain, called the meninges, which is caused by a yeast called *Cryptococcus neoformans* that is inhaled and establishes itself in the lung before being carried by the blood stream to the brain), and even the development of liver cancer through the secretion of a toxin by fungi known as *Aspergillus* that grows on grains or peanuts (called aflatoxin). In the latter case, governmental agencies must monitor the levels of aflatoxins in such products to ensure they are not sold. The situation with yeast meningitis has become even more alarming, in that although it is not a common disease for most of us, it has become so in patients with AIDS (because of their poor immunity) and is one of the four most life-threatening complications of AIDS.

The actinomycetes also represent a large group of microorganisms that descriptively lie midway between the bacteria and the more complex fungi. Found mostly in soil, especially in rich organic environments such as barnyards, some groups grow as branched filaments and produce spores like the fungi, while other groups (which are also found in the soil but in other environments as well, such as in water and various human tissues) resemble bacteria. The importance of this remarkably diverse group of microorganisms lies in their extremes of what we might call "good" and "evil." For the former, almost all the useful antibiotics (more than seventy thus far) are produced by a particular genus of filamentous, soil-inhabiting actinomycete, called *Streptomyces*. The first of them, streptomycin, was discovered in the 1940s by an eminent soil microbiologist, Selman Waksman, who won the Nobel Prize for his concept that such beneficial organisms could exist in the soil. In addition, it was the first successful antibiotic to treat tuberculosis, which ironically is also caused by an actinomycete. Using the royalties obtained from its commercial production, Waksman established the first institute of microbiology in the world, at Rutgers University in 1954 (now known as the Waksman Institute), to study a wide variety of microbiological disciplines. An antibiotic is defined as a substance, produced by a living organism, that can destroy or inhibit the growth of other microorganisms in dilute (or small) concentrations. Why antibiotics are produced naturally in the soil by one particular microorganism is speculative, but they have been of great benefit for the treatment and cure of a multitude of infectious diseases. For over sixty years, this has been the case. Unfortunately, as with the use of any substance that affects bacteria, many resistant mutants have evolved, so now their diseases have become very difficult to treat successfully (we will discuss the problem of resistance to antibiotics further in another chapter). For the latter, two of the most dreaded diseases that have been known since antiquity are caused by bacterial-like actinomycetes; namely, tuberculosis (caused by *Mycobacterium tuberculosis*) and leprosy (caused by *Mycobacterium leprae*). Both pathogens are very different in how they infect and cause their symptoms, yet both can induce a severe inflammation that also damages the host. Tuberculosis will be discussed in a separate chapter.

We have left the "viruses" for last because they cannot be classified as true organisms. The best way to begin is to define what they are in a "descriptive" sense; namely, "a submicroscopic entity capable of being introduced into living cells and of developing there only." This definition stresses (1) that they cannot be visualized in an ordinary light microscope (too small) and (2) that they are inert outside living cells. Virus is the Latin word for "poison." Such is the description of how these obligate, in vivo parasites were first named just before the beginning of the twentieth century by a Dutch microbiologist, Marinus Beijerinck. He added the word "filterable" before "virus" because their activities, such as infecting new cells (he could not see them in the light microscope, as stated above), were still detectable after filtering (removing) all the bacteria from a nutrient solution that then should have been sterile ("pure") but was not. The havoc that viruses inflict on all living organisms (including even bacteria) has been documented in considerable and sometimes vivid detail (in film, for example) throughout the twentieth century and certainly into the twenty-first. They cause an incredible variety of serious and not-so-serious diseases, from the common cold to AIDS, flu (influenza), SARS (severe acute respiratory syndrome), polio, smallpox, yellow fever, newly emerging hemorrhagic fevers (EBOLA), West Nile disease, hepatitis, cold sores (herpes), warts, rabies, mumps, measles, chicken pox, some types of cancer, and on and on. Why? Because they are the ultimate intracellular parasites and because they redirect the metabolism of the cell they infect for their own development. They must do this because by themselves they are not true cells, but simply containers of genetic material surrounded by protective protein coats of great complexity. Thus, they have evolved to use the nutrient-rich inner milieu of a living cell, with all its diversity, to "reproduce" themselves.

Typically, from one infected human cell, literally millions of new viruses can be produced, depending on the virus. However, in some cases, the outcome is not development of the virus but integration (becoming masked or hidden). Incredibly enough, such integration in certain previously harmless bacterial species has spawned diseases such as diphtheria, botulism, and cholera because they carry genetic material that codes for the specific toxin characteristic of the disease. Why "Evolution" has played such a grotesque trick on us is unknown. Although viruses are exceedingly small (usually a hundred times smaller than that of a single bacterial cell, and less than 12,000 times smaller than that of a typical human cell), their shapes and relative sizes are incredible. Some resemble a helix (tobacco mosaic virus), others consist of a "head" and a "tail" (viruses that infect bacteria), and still others are spherical or resemble a polyhedral (polio, HIV, cold virus [Figure 1.6]). These shapes and structures are reflective of the mechanisms used by the virus to attach to the surface of the host cell before passing through into the inner part of the cell, called the cytoplasm.

Before addressing the typical replicative cycle of a virus, we come back to their identity as "living" organisms or not. Certainly, they do not exhibit many of the properties we associate with most living cells; namely, certain cellular structures and the presence of the four macromolecules (both nucleic acids, proteins, carbohydrates, and lipids). Instead, viruses "usually" have only two of the four macromolecules—one nucleic acid and protein—although sometimes their protein coats contain lipids (fats) and carbohydrates as well, and a

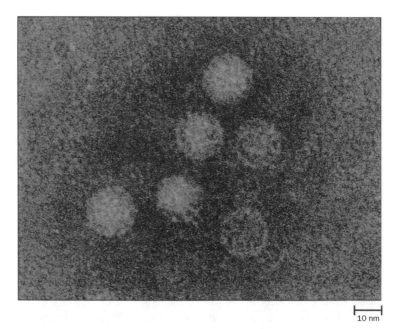

10 nm

FIGURE 1.6 The common cold is caused by a virus, usually a rhinovirus, like the one pictured here. There is no effective vaccine.

multitude of enzymes; in addition, viruses exhibit the generation of and use of the energy of cell metabolism, and adaptation to changing environments. Nevertheless, by virtue of their genetic material, viruses "reproduce" and adapt to changing internal cellular environments by normal evolutionary mechanisms. They are also transmitted to new host cells. Only when they are outside the cell are they inert; they show no typical signs of "life" as we have defined it. Thus, most life scientists consider them to be alive but very simple. I have deliberately not described the chemical composition of the genetic material, which in viruses can exist in one of two forms (DNA or RNA), so that in the next chapter I may discuss them in context with other important aspects of heredity.

All viruses have essentially a similar life cycle, which is very different than that of a normal cell. First, they must be adsorbed on to the surface of the specific cell they infect (Figure 1.7).

There is a remarkable recognition process of attachment that involves specialized "structures" on the protein coat of the virus and "receptor" sites on the cell surface. It is thought by some evolutionists that this great specificity indicates that the virus may have evolved from the cells they infect. Second, the intact virus (usually, but sometimes the genetic material alone) penetrates or is swallowed (almost like the engulfment by a phagocyte or white blood cell) into the host cell, and in a process called "uncoating," the protein layer is removed from the viral genetic material by special enzymes contained within

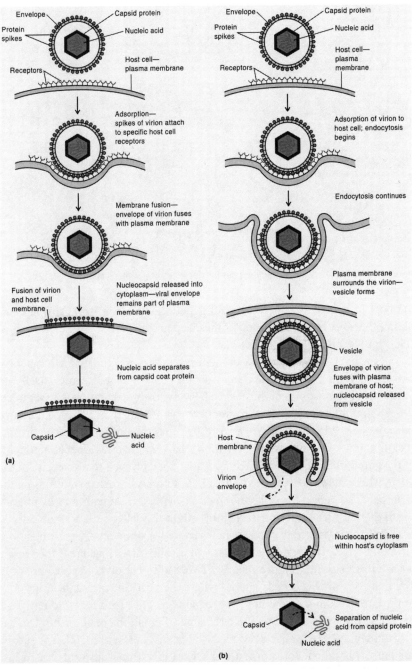

FIGURE 1.7 Entry of enveloped animal viruses into host cells: (a) entry following membrane fusion and (b) entry by endocytosis (a process by which the host cell actually engulfs the virus). (See Plate 4)

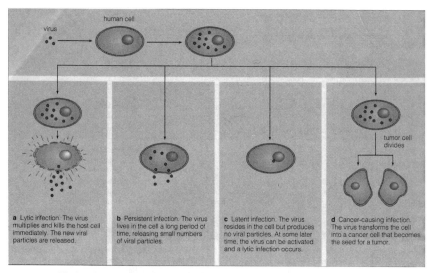

FIGURE 1.8 Viral pathogenesis. The four possible outcomes of a viral infection.

the host or the virus. Once the viral genetic material is "free" in the cytoplasm, there are four possible outcomes, depending on the virus and the host cell (Figure 1.8).

In the most typical outcome of higher cells, the viral genetic material must pass through the cytoplasm and into the nucleus, where it integrates itself into one of the chromosomes of the host cell. From this protected site, it first directs the cell to synthesize new viral components, which are then assembled to produce the new "virion." The process is called maturation. In effect, the process is akin to that of an automobile assembly plant, where individual components of the automobile are constructed and then are conveyed to a final site in the plant, where they are assembled into a new automobile. After maturation, the virus particles depart the cell either by destroying it from within or by migrating to the cell surface, where they "bud" off. In this latter situation the cells do not "die" but are forced to produce new virions for some time, a truly insidious viral "directive." The first type of infection is called "lytic," whereas the second is called "persistent" (Figure 1.8a, b). Two additional outcomes are possible. The first (or third) is called "latent," where the virus integrates itself into one of the chromosomes of the host but remains inactive (produces no new viral particles) until it is activated at a later time (if at all; the relationship can last indefinitely), whereby a lytic process usually ensues (Figure 1.8c). The second (or fourth) is called "transformation," where the virus is also integrated into one or more of the chromosomes but ultimately induces the cell to become transformed into a cancer cell (Figure 1.8d). There are many examples of these four striking outcomes in the virus "kingdom." Some will be discussed in special chapters concerning a specific disease.

2

Fundamental Concepts of Biology and Chemistry Help Understand Pathogenicity

A. Genetics: The Nature of the Gene and Its Chemical Structure (DNA)

Throughout our discussion thus far, direct and indirect references to genetic phenomena have been made either for pathogens or their hosts. These include the use of terms and phrases such as "mutation," "adaptation," "natural selection," "genetic defect," "phase variation," "auxotroph," "genes," "DNA and RNA," "chromosome," "enzyme synthesis," and "feedback loop" to try to explain a specific phenomenon. But have we really explained what is meant by such "genetic phenomena"? Not really. Thus, this section will, I hope, provide a brief overview of the meaning of this important phrase as well as illustrate how they apply generally and specifically to microorganisms, especially pathogens (including viruses). First of all, the term "genetics" is defined as the biological study of heredity (or the inheritance of various traits and their variation from one generation to the next). How does that definition help us understand "genetic phenomena"? A great deal, because these traits are inherited under the control of physical components called genes, which are organized sequentially on structures called chromosomes, found only in the nucleus of all living cells. However, right here there is a fundamental difference between "higher" cells, which we call "eukaryotic," and bacteria, which we call "prokaryotic," because the latter do not contain true nuclei. This presented a problem to early microbiologists, who thought they did not have "genes." This hypothesis was overturned only eventually by many studies during the latter part of the twentieth century, starting in the 1940s with the founding of the field of microbial genetics and its sister field, molecular biology. Perhaps the most remarkable aspect in the entire history of modern genetics is that experiments with those "Johnny come lately" microorganisms led to the initial elucidation of the chemical composition of the gene, as well as indicating how such genes expressed their control of inheritance and other aspects of cell function. Both these classic experiments were accomplished well before understanding how the particular chemical composing the gene carried out its remarkable functions. Of course, this "chemical" is DNA (or deoxyribonucleic acid), but ever since it was discovered in 1869 by a brilliant German chemist, Frederick Meischer (who himself succumbed to tuberculosis at the age of fifty-two), it was not thought to be of importance in heredity, even though it was found primarily in the nucleus of higher cells as well as in sperm cells. Then, in 1944 three scientists at the Rockefeller Institute, O. Avery, C. MacLeod, and M. McCarty, reinvestigated an interesting observation made sixteen years previously by F. Griffith in England, working with the dreaded pathogen that caused pneumonia (*Streptococcus pneumoniae*).

Griffith observed that "pneumococci" (for short) could cause pneumonia in mice only if they were surrounded by a capsule that inhibited phagocytosis by white blood cells in the mice (one of the virulence factors we discussed previously). When pneumococci without capsules (mutants) were injected into mice, they survived. Griffith next inoculated mice with a mixture of live, noncapsulated pneumococci and heat-killed (dead), capsulated pneumococci to see whether some property of the pneumococci could "transform" the noncapsulated pneumococci and make them pathogenic. To Griffith's great surprise, the experiment worked, in that pneumococci isolated from dead or dying mice were fully capsulated, and they remained so from then on; they were as pathogenic as any capsulated pneumococcus. Yet, heat-killed, capsulated pneumococci injected by themselves into mice did no damage. In an attempt to duplicate these in vivo results with more-painstaking in vitro analysis, the three Rockefeller scientists, after many years, isolated the transforming principle (Figure 2.1), which turned out to be DNA. They added purified DNA extracted from encapsulated pneumococci to cultures of non-capsulated pneumococci and were able to recover fully capsulated pneumococci, which when injected into mice caused pneumonia. Somehow the DNA was incorporated into the noncapsulated cells and carried genetic information to induce them to synthesize a capsule. How was still a mystery, but it was the first direct evidence that the organic chemical DNA carried genetic information!

The other classic experiment that provided significant insights into how genes functioned was accomplished by two scientists, George Beadle and Edward Tatum, in 1941 (for which they eventually won the Nobel Prize). Working with the fungus *Neurospora crasa*, a common bread mold, they demonstrated indirectly that genes control the synthesis of enzymes (which are proteins). Their experiment led to the formulation of one of the great principles of modern genetics, the "one-gene, one-enzyme" hypothesis, which had to be modified only slightly, as described in section C of this chapter. They first cultured the fungus in a very simple growth solution (medium), called

Organisms injected	Results

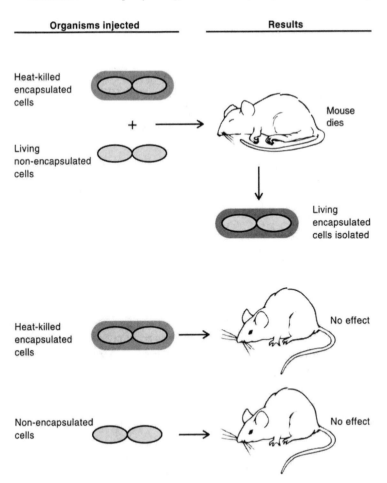

Heat-killed encapsulated cells

Living non-encapsulated cells

Mouse dies

Living encapsulated cells isolated

Heat-killed encapsulated cells — No effect

Non-encapsulated cells — No effect

FIGURE 2.1 Demonstration of the transforming principle.

"minimal" because it contained just a sugar compound for deriving energy and mineral salts. They then exposed the fungal growth to X-rays, which were known even then to affect genes by changing or damaging them. A number of the resultant mutants they isolated were unable to grow in the simple medium unless they contained preformed nutrients such as mixtures of B vitamins or amino acids. This result suggested to Beadle and Tatum that the specific gene that was altered could no longer be functional in supplying one of the specific nutrients in these mixtures. Further intensive analysis revealed which of the vitamins or which of the amino acids (there are twenty of them) was required by the mutant. They concluded that the gene present in that particular mutant was defective in controlling the synthesis of an enzyme required to supply the missing nutrient.

B. Metabolism Consists of Chemical Reactions, without Which Life Would Not Exist

Why enzymes? For this question we have to digress and discuss the nature of cell metabolism. All living cells maintain their existence and perform their functions (whatever they are) by chemical reactions. Without chemical reactions there is no life. The sum of all chemical reactions carried out by living cells is encompassed in the term "metabolism." Metabolism is divided into two major classes: those chemical reactions that produce chemical energy (derived from the decomposition primarily of organic compounds such as carbohydrates and fats), and those chemical reactions that use the energy for the synthesis of cell structures and other components that characterize the cell's function (derived from basic building blocks such as amino acids, purines and pyrimidines, and fatty acids). The former chemical reaction is called "catabolism," while the latter is called "anabolism." Each process is intimately linked, and there are literally thousands of reactions controlled very carefully and precisely so that the cell does not "wear out." Metabolic reactions occur in a sequence that is called a metabolic pathway. The sequence itself is characterized by the production of a series of intermediate chemical compounds, starting from the initial one, which is gradually altered chemically until the final end product is produced. Why are there so many "intermediate" reactions and why cannot the initial compound be transformed in one step to "save" wear and tear? The reason for this slow progression lies in the fact that a significant amount of heat is generated by each chemical reaction, which could damage and ultimately kill the cell unless it is produced in small amounts so that the cell can dissipate it. The cell would be destroyed instantly if the chemical reaction that changed the initial substrate to the final product occurred in one step! Thus, each intermediate chemical reaction results in the release of small "packets" of energy and heat. The former is saved during some reactions for synthetic purposes and to help drive the pathway to the next intermediate, while the latter is dissipated.

C. Biological Catalysts (Enzymes) Mediate Every Chemical Reaction in the Cell

By now you probably have guessed (but if not, I will inform you) that every one of these chemical reactions is mediated by a different enzyme, which loosely defined are biological catalysts (Figure 2.2).

They act by controlling the rate and extent of converting one chemical compound (the substrate) to another (the product), without being altered themselves. How they accomplish this amazing feat is beyond the scope of this text, but what better way is there for genes to control the functioning of a cell

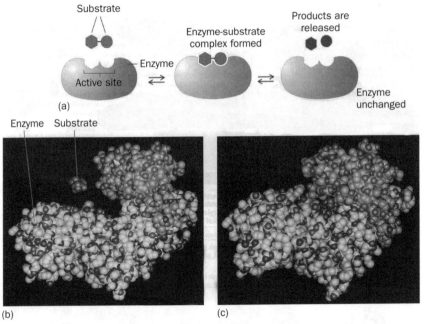

FIGURE 2.2 Mechanism of enzyme action: (a) The substrate binds to the active site, forming an enzyme-substrate complex. The products are then released, leaving the enzyme unchanged and free to combine with new substrate molecules. (b) A model showing an enzyme and its substrate. (c) The binding of the substrate to the active site causes the shape of the flexible enzyme to change slightly. (See Plate 5)

than by controlling the synthesis and expression of enzymes, the "one-gene, one-enzyme" hypothesis that Beadle and Tatum first proposed. However, since there are proteins, which are not enzymatic but structural, the phrase has been changed to "one gene, one protein."

D. Genes Control the Synthesis and Expression of Enzymes (Which Are Proteins) and Hence Control the Functioning of the Cell

The two classic experiments described in section A of this chapter were instrumental after a while in greatly stimulating other life scientists to ask the all-important "how." How does the gene control the synthesis of enzymes? How does the actual metabolic process unfold? How does the gene store its genetic information, which is DNA, to specify so many thousands of proteins? How does the gene duplicate itself? And for our purposes, how do all these questions relate to an understanding of pathogenicity? In one of the greatest insights of modern biological endeavor, the structure of this master macromolecule of the cell DNA was elucidated by two future Nobel Prize winners, James Watson and

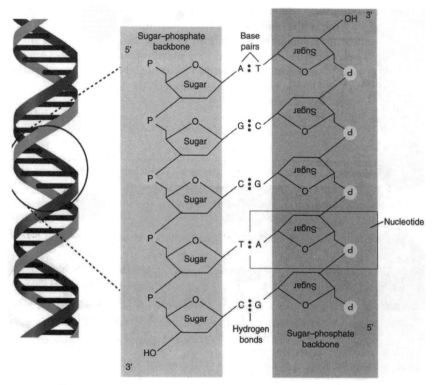

FIGURE 2.3 The double helix of DNA. The two strands of DNA are antiparallel; one strand is oriented to the 5' to 3' direction, and its complement is oriented in the 3' to 5' direction. Hydrogen bonding occurs between the complementary base pairs; three bonds form between a G-C base pair, and two bonds form between an A-T base pair. (See Plate 6)

Francis Crick, who published their short paper in 1953 in the scientific journal *Nature* (Watson and Crick 1953), titled "Molecular structure of nucleic acids: A structure for deoxyribose nucleic acid" (*Nature*, 171, 1953: 737–738) (Figure 2.3).

In one master stroke, the structure could explain (1) how the genetic information was stored, and (2) how it could be duplicated precisely from generation to generation. The third insight—namely, how the structure controlled cell function (gene expression)—had to wait for new discoveries that elucidated the actual mechanisms and what small and large molecules and structures were involved. Basically, DNA consists of a long thread of four basic compounds called nucleotides (adenine, guanine, cytosine, and thymine; we also call them "bases") that are linked together in an endless variable sequence, but a sequence that is programmed by evolution. Watson and Crick proposed that each gene on a molecular level consists of a certain defined number of these four bases in a particular sequence. In other words, genes differ by virtue of their differences in sequence of the four bases, as well as variations in length. Watson and Crick also proposed that in the cell, DNA exists as a double helix, one helical strand wrapped around another. If each strand were unwound and separated, the structure would resemble a ladder, with the sides of the ladder made up of the same portion of each of the four nucleotides (sugar and phosphate), while the "rungs" of the ladder consist of that portion of the nucleotide that confers its specificity as a different base (two different purines, adenine or guanine; or two different pyrimidines, thymine or cytosine). What is more amazing is that the two strands are complementary. By that is meant whatever unique portion of the nucleotide sticks out inwardly from one strand to make up half the rung of the ladder will determine what unique portion of the nucleotide sticks out inwardly from the other strand. Thus, for every adenine in one strand, only a thymine can bind to it from the other strand; similarly for a cytosine and guanine. Thus, in a sense the sequence of bases in one strand determines the sequence of bases in the other one. Exact duplication of the double helix could occur in the cell, the two scientists reasoned, by (1) unwinding each helix and (2) using the separated strands as templates to direct (via enzymes) the assembly of its complementary strand, which would consist of one original strand and one newly synthesized strand. Once synthesis (which we call semiconservative) and rewinding of the new double helix are complete, one of them would be transferred to a daughter cell by cell division. In fact, with the incredible coordination of many different enzymes and other proteins (over forty have been identified in bacteria alone, now termed a "replisome"), this is exactly how replication (or the faithful transfer) of the gene pool occurs from one generation to the next. Moreover, it does not take a "rocket scientist" to envision how a mistake in the gene can occur, altering it for better or worse and resulting in a mutation. Simply by altering one base in the sequence of the gene, a different sequence is produced. This is exactly what happened in the experiments of Beadle and Tatum, who, by exposing the DNA of the fungus to X-rays (as discussed previously), altered the sequence of a particular gene in a specific metabolic pathway supplying an important amino acid or vitamin. Of course, the major problem is how the information in the sequence of four bases in DNA is expressed in a specific protein consisting of twenty amino acids, also in a variable sequence.

E. The Mechanism of Protein Synthesis Involves a Complex Series of Metabolic Reactions and Cellular Organelles, Starting with DNA, a Related Macromolecule (RNA), and the Ribosome (the Protein-Synthesizing Factory)

Simply put, the four bases in DNA act as a chemical code that somehow is translated to code for the twenty-odd amino acids in a protein. However, if one base is responsible for one amino acid, that can signify only four amino acids. Even a two-base sequence is insufficient, since all the variations of a two-base code could signify only sixteen amino acids. Therefore, by necessity, a three-base sequence was the obvious solution because all combinations of this sequence could signify sixty-four amino acids, far more than required. In fact, this "genetic code" (as it is now called) is universal; that is, it exists in all living organisms and is mostly the same in each of them—no matter the species! Thus, a specific sequence of three bases, which are now designated as codons, specifies one amino acid, which in turn is linked to other amino acids that have been designated by other codons in sequence to form a specific protein. This implies that a gene must be long enough (at least three times longer in terms of its base sequence) to code for a specific protein. It also must contain information (in terms of specific sequences) as to where the coding region of the gene begins (for the protein) and where it ends. Of course, many important problems remained to be solved, such as which codon specified which amino acid and what did the excess codons specify? For example, were some of them redundant—that is, could several codons code for the same amino acid? Were there codons that specified no amino acids (to signal the end of a specific protein)? Was there a specific codon that specified the first amino acid in a protein? And, the big "enchilada," how did the process actually occur in the cell, where did it occur, and how was it controlled? It took years to answer all these questions, and there are still many details being elucidated.

Nevertheless, the basic outline of gene expression—there are two separate but interrelated biochemical processes involved—is as follows (Figures 2.4, 2.5).

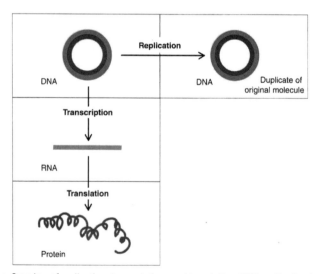

FIGURE 2.4 Overview of replication, transcription, and translation. DNA replication is the process that duplicates DNA, so that its encoded information can be passed on to future generations. Transcription is the process that copies the genetic information into a transitional form, RNA. Translation is the process that deciphers the encoded information to synthesize a specific protein. (See Plate 7)

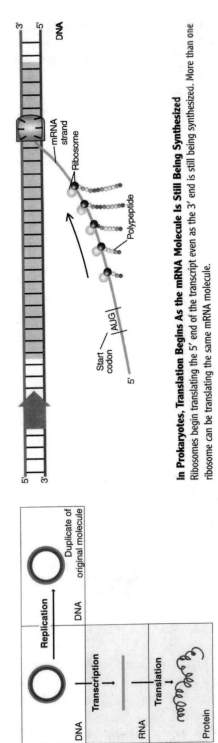

In Prokaryotes, Translation Begins As the mRNA Molecule Is Still Being Synthesized
Ribosomes begin translating the 5′ end of the transcript even as the 3′ end is still being synthesized. More than one ribosome can be translating the same mRNA molecule.

FIGURE 2.5 In prokaryotes, translation begins as the mRNA molecule is still being synthesized. Ribosomes begin translating the 5′ end of the transcript even as the 3′ end is still being synthesized. More than one ribosome can be translating the same mRNA molecule. (See Plate 8)

The first process is called "transcription," in which a macromolecule very similar to DNA, called RNA (or ribonucleic acid), is synthesized (or transcribed) by an enzyme called RNA polymerase under the direction of one of the strands of DNA, to produce a complementary single-stranded RNA macromolecule that is the exact length of the specific gene being expressed (including start and stop sites). Thus, whatever the base sequence is of the "director" DNA strand, the base sequence of the RNA strand will be identical to that of the other DNA strand (with a minor substitution of one base uracil in RNA for thymine in DNA). This RNA is called messenger RNA or mRNA because it contains the exact information (the transcript) encoded in one of the DNA strands [also termed the (+) strand]. The other DNA strand, the "director" or template strand, is called the (−) strand. In some cases, the mRNA can contain information for a number of genes of a particular metabolic pathway, since the genes themselves are adjacent to each other on the chromosome, especially in bacteria, which have only one chromosome. It is appropriate to point out here that RNA too can contain genetic information, storing the code in its sequence of bases. In fact, many deadly viruses, such as HIV and influenza, use RNA alone as their chromosome. The only chemical difference between the two is that uracil (a pyrimidine) replaces thymine in RNA, and there is a slightly different sugar molecule in the latter as well. It sounds complicated, but if you illustrate and name the strands by yourself, using specific base sequences for both strands and mRNA as a model, the process will become clearer. The second process is called "translation," an extremely complicated but remarkable process in which the genetic information in the form of the base sequence codons on the mRNA transcript is uncoded to synthesize the protein (Figure 2.6).

The protein itself is built up by adding each of the twenty amino acids one by one, starting with the first one (which in bacteria is always the same, a slightly modified amino acid called "formyl" methionine, whose codon, by the way, is adenine-thymine [uracil in RNA]—guanine or "AUG" for short). Gradually, a chain of chemically linked amino acids (or a peptide) is produced that, as it extends in length, results in a polypeptide and then finally in the complete protein. Many components are required for the conversion of the codons into a protein. The main ones consist of two additional RNA macromolecules besides mRNA, called "ribosomal" RNA (rRNA) and a relatively small-species RNA called "transfer" RNA (tRNA), as well as numerous control factors and enzymes plus a cellular structure where all the components come together in an "intimate" fashion, called a "ribosome" or the protein-synthesizing factory of the cell. There are literally thousands of ribosomes in each bacterial cell, which are composed of many proteins bound to two types of ribosomal RNAs involved in the conversion.

The first step is the enzymatic attachment of each amino acid to one of twenty types of tRNA, one for each amino acid. How does the enzyme "know"

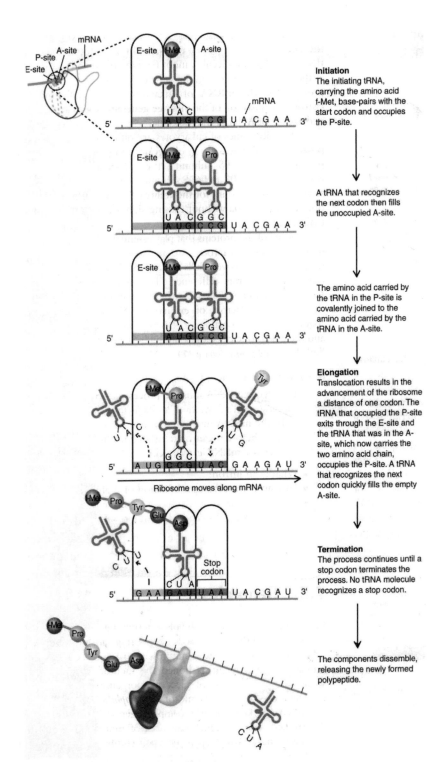

Initiation
The initiating tRNA, carrying the amino acid f-Met, base-pairs with the start codon and occupies the P-site.

A tRNA that recognizes the next codon then fills the unoccupied A-site.

The amino acid carried by the tRNA in the P-site is covalently joined to the amino acid carried by the tRNA in the A-site.

Elongation
Translocation results in the advancement of the ribosome a distance of one codon. The tRNA that occupied the P-site exits through the E-site and the tRNA that was in the A-site, which now carries the two amino acid chain, occupies the P-site. A tRNA that recognizes the next codon quickly fills the empty A-site.

Termination
The process continues until a stop codon terminates the process. No tRNA molecule recognizes a stop codon.

The components dissemble, releasing the newly formed polypeptide.

FIGURE 2.6 The process of translation. (See Plate 9)

which amino acid attaches to which tRNA? There are a number of signals, but the main one is a sequence of three bases in the middle of the tRNA (of about seventy nucleotides) that is the exact complement of the codon in the mRNA transcript for that particular amino acid. These are called "anticodons." Thus, the anticodon for the amino acid "formyl" methionine (mentioned above), whose codon is AUG, would be UAC. The tRNA–amino acid complex is called "charged," and it "migrates" to the ribosome, where it "meets" the mRNA with its codons. Both of them have special sites on the ribosome where they bind temporarily, with the mRNA moving across the top of the ribosome (like swiping a credit card through a slot) and the first charged tRNA binding, also temporarily, to one of two grooves in the ribosome, called "P" (the left one), and leaving the right groove (called "A") open. These two grooves lie right beneath the mRNA binding sites. Now, picture the dynamics of the process if you can. As the first codon (AUG) from the mRNA transcript starts its journey along the top of the ribosome, it temporarily complexes with the anticodon (UAC) of the charged methionine tRNA that has been induced to move into "P" groove. It is the only one that can bind there, for reasons not completely understood even today. The methionine is bound to the end of the tRNA at the bottom of the groove. Next, the codon-anticodon complex is dissociated, and the mRNA moves past the first groove and keeps on moving over the second "A" groove. Another charged tRNA will be induced to settle into that groove, depending on what the second codon is after the AUG codon. Let us assume it is UUU (which is the codon specifying the amino acid named phenylalanine). Thus, the only charged tRNA that can be induced to move into the "A" groove and bind there is one containing the anticodon AAA, which will temporarily complex with the UUU codon from the moving mRNA transcript. Its attached amino acid (phenylalanine) will now be placed adjacent to the first amino acid methionine at the bottom of the "A" groove.

Now you may sense what is transpiring. The two amino acids (methionine and phenylalanine) adjacent to each other at the bottom of each groove will be chemically linked by an enzyme that is part of the ribosome to form a dipeptide. At the same time the first tRNA will be disattached from its amino acid (methionine), which is a signal for the tRNA to be removed from its "P" groove by passing through an exit groove called "E" and leaving the ribosome. This departure, in turn, provides another signal in which an amazing reaction occurs, whereby the second charged tRNA from the "A" groove together with its two bound amino acids is "translocated" into the "P" groove, leaving the "A" groove empty. Of course, while all this is transpiring, the mRNA transcript continues to move along the top of the ribosome, now positioning the third codon above the vacant "A" groove. Let us say the codon is UCA, which specifies the amino acid named serine. This signifies that the charged tRNA settling into that groove will contain the anticodon AGU, with serine at the bottom of the groove. The same process as described above will then ensue: the dipeptide from the tRNA in the "P" groove will bind to serine to form a "tripeptide," with the tRNA in the "P" groove becoming disattached by passing through the "E" groove and being removed from the ribosome. This will then be followed by another translocation of the tripeptide-charged tRNA complex from the "A" groove to the "P" groove, leaving the "A" groove vacant once again. Thus, in time, a protein will be formed, one amino acid at a time. However, the most important concept to understand and appreciate from this incredible two-step process of gene expression is that the long polypeptide chain of amino acids that results in a specific protein is produced as specified by the codon sequence in the mRNA transcript, which in turn was specified by the (-) template strand of DNA. Thus, the "one-gene, one-protein" hypothesis is confirmed and completed!

Now that you have congratulated yourself on understanding how one gene controls the synthesis of one protein, we can move on to a relatively new metabolic process that was uncovered a while back, first in animal cells and then in bacteria and even viruses, which amazingly resulted in one gene controlling the synthesis of more than one protein. Not only that, but the process revealed that RNA, besides acting as a message from DNA (m-RNA), as an amino acid carrier (t-RNA), or as being part of the ribosome (r-RNA), can also act as an enzyme (called a ribozyme). Such ribozymes are involved in what is termed "gene splicing." They cut or "splice" the m-RNA that has originally faithfully copied the base sequence in DNA into smaller m-RNA segments, which are then rejoined to form different "species" of m-RNA. These then can code for more than one protein. Thus, gene control of protein synthesis has evolved in a myriad of ways to provide the "most bang for the buck"; that is, the production of a diversity of proteins much greater than defined, simply by the sequence of bases that make up the gene.

F. Gene Expression is Tightly Regulated to Economize and Preserve Cell Integrity

The amazing process of how a protein is synthesized represents just the beginning of gene expression because of the many controls that exist to determine (1) when the gene is expressed, (2) under what environmental circumstances, and (3) when and how expression ceases. For microorganisms (including pathogens), there are a variety of special considerations. First of all, because they are "single"-celled organisms directly exposed to a constantly changing outside environment (no protection like "skin" or a buffering circulatory systems in a multicellular organism, like "us"), they must be equipped to adapt to them rapidly. Secondly, because microorganisms have only one set of genes organized linearly on one chromosome that has very few protective components to shield it from internal (cytoplasmic) or external (physical or

chemical) stresses, they must be able to repair any damage to a gene or genes rapidly, as well as to grow rapidly to provide new gene "reservoirs." Third, microorganisms must not "wear out" while gene expression is occurring. That is, since the processes of transcription and translation require considerable levels of energy, microorganisms must be able to "repress" those genes that are not needed and to express only those that are. Thus, the energy that is "saved" can be used to synthesize other products that maximize growth rates. As a result, microorganisms have evolved a striking ability to regulate expression of specific genes in a metabolic pathway in response to small changes in the environment (much more so than higher eukaryotic cells). Gene expression is turned on when certain nutrient substrates are available so that the protein products of these genes can be synthesized, and it is turned off when the substrates are no longer available or the gene products are no longer required. We have already described one such "turn on and turn off" capability that pathogens use to sequester scarce iron. It involves a combination of increased toxin synthesis to destroy susceptible host cells that then release "free" iron, followed by sequestering it in complexes called siderophores, which are also synthesized as a result of gene expression. When the levels of free iron decrease, somehow this acts as a feedback signal to "turn off" the genes that are being expressed to synthesize toxin. Nevertheless, it should be recognized that there are some important genes controlling the expression of certain metabolic pathways that are always functioning to maintain basic life processes (such as DNA synthesis, tRNA and rRNA synthesis and secretion). They are called "housekeeping" (or constitutive) genes.

Basically, most mechanisms for the control of gene expression operate at the levels of transcription and translation. Some others related to those major ones include mechanisms that affect the stability or processing of the mRNA transcript, the further processing of the protein after translation, and the function of the protein itself. However, the largest impact on gene expression in bacteria is at the level of transcription, or the "beginning." It is a fact, as we stated above, that many types of metabolic pathways do not function except when they are needed, which implies that transcription of the genes in those pathways is "shut off" like a light switch. The question is what turns on the switch? Early studies in the 1930s by the Swedish scientist Karström focused on small sugar molecules present in the environment that stimulated the production of enzymes that degraded them chemically (for catabolic purposes). The phenomenon was termed "adaptive" enzyme synthesis. However, when it was recognized much later (beginning in the 1950s) that genes controlled the synthesis of enzymes (as we have discussed extensively previously), it was difficult to understand what role these small molecules played in gene expression. This "conundrum" was finally resolved in a series of brilliant genetic and biochemical experiments in the 1960s, primarily by French scientists, notably J. Monod, F. Jacob, A. Lwoff, and E. Wollman at the Pasteur Institute in

Paris (for which Jacob and Monod later won the Nobel Prize). It was one of the highlights of microbial genetics in its early years and provided the spark for many further investigations into how genetic control of gene expression in bacteria was influenced by the availability (or not) of small molecules in the internal or external environment. After many insightful experiments, they devised a model that encompassed all their observations, called the "operon" (Figure 2.7).

The operon was a genetic unit of regulation for a series of genes involved in expressing enzymes for a particular metabolic pathway. It consisted of two types of genes, "structural" and "regulatory." The structural genes coded for the specific enzymes in the pathway and were physically located on the

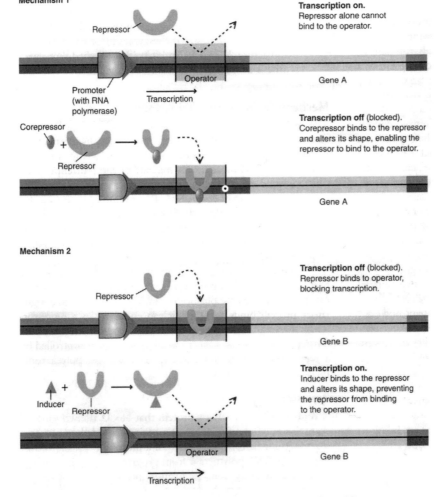

FIGURE 2.7 Transcriptional regulation by repressors (the operon). (See Plate 10)

chromosome adjacent to each other in sequence (that is, the first gene coding for the first enzyme, the second gene coding for the second enzyme, etc.). The regulatory gene (usually only one) did code for a protein that was expressed by transcription and translation, called the "repressor." It was not an enzyme and was not adjacent to the structural genes but was located some distance away on the chromosome. This repressor protein (unique for each operon) prevented transcription of the structural genes, by binding tightly to a region before the beginning of the first gene in the metabolic pathway, known as the operator region, where the enzyme that would normally initiate the synthesis of mRNA (RNA polymerase) also binds. Under these conditions, the RNA polymerase was sterically prevented from attaching to its DNA substrate. Why was it necessary only for the repressor protein to bind to the beginning of the first gene? Would not the remaining genes of the pathway still require repressor binding as well to prevent their transcriptions? The answer lies in economy of expression. That is, in most metabolic pathways of this type, once the first gene is "turned on" by binding RNA polymerase (see below), transcription "reads through" all the other genes sequentially with one long mRNA transcript, thus negating the requirement for multiple RNA polymerase molecules and multiple repressor molecules to inhibit their binding. The long mRNA is called a "polycistronic" message. As pointed out above, this is the usual case of negative control of gene expression. However, the brilliant insight of the French scientists involved unraveling how the small substrate exerted its role in "adaptive" enzyme synthesis. They proposed that it did not affect the synthesis of any one enzyme directly, but rather that it had the propensity to bind to the repressor, which caused a change in the conformation (shape) of its physical structure (called an allosteric change), resulting in an inability to bind to the beginning of the first gene. In turn, this inability permitted RNA polymerase to bind to the gene to initiate transcription of the structural genes, thus "inducing" the synthesis of all the enzymes of that particular metabolic pathway. Actually, there are other small molecules resembling the small substrate chemically and structurally that are not metabolized by the enzymes of the pathway, which can also bind to the repressor and inactivate it. Thus, this phenomenon of "derepression" of the metabolic pathway is called "induction," and the small molecule is called an "inducer." It should be further pointed out that many repressor proteins for different inducible metabolic pathways have been detected and purified, and they have been shown to bind to the beginning of the first gene of their respective metabolic pathways.

There are, as one might expect, many ramifications and a number of modifications of this genetic control mechanism for gene expression. For example, mutations in a number of genes in the operon, such as the repressor gene that produces a "defective" repressor protein, or the first structural gene that prevents a normal repressor protein from binding, can cause a fundamental change from an "inducible" to a "constitutive" operon, where the particular metabolic pathway would always be operative, regardless of whether the inducer was present or not. In contrast, there is a class of operons that exist normally as a constitutive genetic control unit where the repressor is inactive and must be ultimately activated. Many of these latter types involve the synthesis of amino acids, which must be available in growing cells even in an environment devoid of them, to supply building blocks for ongoing protein synthesis. Thus, the first gene in such an operon binds RNA polymerase to initiate transcription of the structural genes coding for enzymes involved in the synthesis of the specific amino acid. Many such operons have between five and seven structural genes. With time, a significant amount of the end-product amino acid will accumulate and be available for translation. However, its continued accumulation becomes counterproductive, wasting energy. In a remarkable example of "feedback" control, the excess amino acid, which is called a "corepressor," binds to the inactive repressor protein, changing its conformation and causing it to bind to the beginning of the first structural gene of the operon. As in the inducible systems, the binding inhibits the ability of RNA polymerase to attach to its DNA substrate, effectively shutting down gene expression. If the amino acid is already available as a nutrient in the environment, it will act as a corepressor in the same way. As a general rule, many inducible operons involve catabolism of different energy sources, since they are needed only when such sources are available in the environment. In contrast, as indicated above, many repressible "end product" operons involve anabolism of building blocks or precursors, since they are needed regardless of whether the precursor is present in the environment or not. Although there are still other types of control mechanisms that affect gene expression, such as "positive" ones, which, for example, act to stimulate the binding of RNA polymerase to its DNA substrate, we have to stop somewhere and begin to discuss how they affect pathogenicity. Suffice it to say, as stated in the beginning of this section, that microorganisms exhibit an incredible array of controls for gene expression and its "fine tuning" so that they can adapt to a myriad of rapidly changing environments. For pathogens, such control is essential to express their virulence factors.

G. Genetic Modifications in the Process of Gene Expression in Microbes Are Varied and Complex. They Include Mutations, Transfer Transformation (Recombination) of Genes from One Cell to Another, and Many Other Variations of These Events

Now that we have a general understanding of the nature of genes, how they work, and how their expression is controlled in bacteria, we can begin to elaborate on references made previously to genetic phenomena in discussing various aspects of pathogenicity. Nevertheless, we should not lose sight of the fact that in "real life" the DNA components of the gene are packed tightly in the bacterial cell, which when treated in a certain way chemically can burst out of the cell to reveal how huge the entire DNA macromolecule is, and how daunting the complexities of its interactions must be (Figure 2.8).

With this appreciation, we can turn to terms such as "mutation," "auxotroph," and "genetic defect," which all refer to a change in the base sequence of a particular gene that must involve a change in a codon either spontaneously or after exposure to some deleterious physical or chemical agent (Figure 2.9). In turn, this codon will code for a different amino acid (all it takes is one), resulting in a change in a specific protein. For example, a change in the middle base from "U" in the codon UUA that codes for leucine to "C" will yield a different codon, UCA, which will code for serine.

Interestingly enough, the change can occur in a part of the protein that does not affect its function (sometimes called cryptic), but if it does (such as the binding site of an enzyme to its substrate), the effect can be profound, such as in an auxotrophic mutant. As was described previously, this type of mutant requires a particular nutrient preformed in order to grow because the mutation occurred in one of the enzymes involved in synthesizing it (such as an amino acid or purine and pyrimidine). In the case of a type of mouse typhoid that is caused by a purine-requiring auxotroph, such a phenomenon is responsible for the amelioration of the disease if the purine is present at low levels. However, strictly speaking, whether a mutation is harmful or beneficial to the specific pathogen (or any organism) depends on the environment. Will it provide a selective advantage such as in a number of pathogens we discussed

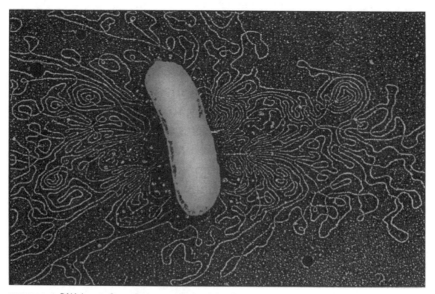

FIGURE 2.8 DNA bursts from the treated bacterial cell.

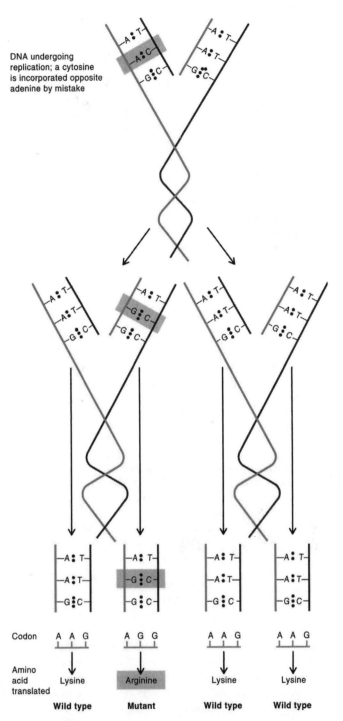

FIGURE 2.9 Base substitution. Shown here is the generation of a mutant organism as a result of the incorporation of a pyrimidine base (cytosine) in place of thymine in DNA replication. (See Plate 11)

(such as scarlet fever and perhaps even AIDS; viruses too are subject to mutations) that have become accommodated to their host, allowing both to survive longer? More directly, will the mutation allow a pathogen to become resistant to a specific antibiotic? Thus, "genetic defect" is perhaps the wrong phrase to use to define a mutation. Rather, a mutation is defined as a spontaneous and undirected change in the genetic makeup of an organism, which geneticists call the genotype, and that allows it to express a new trait, which is called the phenotype. The environment will determine whether the mutation will survive or not. Of course, there are mutations such as those in "housekeeping" genes that are lethal and where a selective "environment" plays little role.

Another phenomenon discussed previously, "phase variation," cannot be considered a mutation because it occurs too quickly, but it does alter gene expression and does affect virulence. The phenomenon involves the random switching on and off of certain genes, such as those coding for surface proteins on particular pathogens. How this occurs is beyond the scope of our discussion, but it permits some pathogens to escape the immune response because the shift occurs in those proteins that antibodies (the proteins generated by the immune system, which takes time to produce) must bind to in order to begin the process of destruction. However, if different surface proteins are present, the original antibodies are useless and new ones must be generated again. What about "other" genetic phenomena? If you recall, two of them, which were described in a previous section, expand the "adaptability" of pathogens greatly and focus not on an internal change in the organism's genes, described above (mutation followed by selection), but on "fresh" insertions of new genetic material. Such insertions can catapult a potential pathogen to "new" heights of virulence. However, in addition, these "enrichments" have shown that one of the major sources of genetic variation, which in higher organisms involves "sexual" reproduction, can also occur in microorganisms. The scientific term for this activity is called "recombination," which is generally defined as "an exchange or reassortment of chromosomes or their parts contributed by both parents that brings about new combinations of genes by the process of integration or crossing over." Such new genic combinations can provide tremendous flexibility to any organism in response to rapidly changing environmental conditions.

Furthermore, there is little doubt that these two cornerstones of evolution, mutation and selection, as well as recombination, have contributed profoundly either to newly emerging or reemerging pathogenic types to which we humans must also adapt. The first one referred to previously (see Figure 2.1) involves transformation, by which "naked" DNA (or part of its chromosome) derived from one strain of a particular species is incorporated by another member of that species and then integrated into the chromosome of the recipient by recombination. This recombination event confers new traits (or phenotypes) upon the latter, which it did not possess previously. In the example cited, nonpathogenic pneumococci (the cause of pneumonia) were transformed with DNA derived from pathogenic pneumococci, rendering the former pathogenic by virtue of being able to form a capsule that protects them from phagocytosis. The second one involves recombination by an intact bacterial virus, by which the infecting virus does not undergo the typical developmental life cycle of producing hundreds of new viruses but instead integrates its chromosome into that of its host by recombination and becomes masked or hidden, multiplying once per generation as part of the host's chromosome. In the example cited previously, harmless bacterial species became dangerous pathogens because the viral chromosome contained genes coding for deadly toxins such as diphtheria, botulism, or cholera. We call such bacteria "lysogens," and their acquisition of these new deadly traits is termed "lysogenic conversion." However, there is another type of recombination event mediated by bacterial viruses (also called a bacteriophage or phage) termed "transduction" (generalized or specialized), which can also create a new pathogen from a harmless strain (Figures 2.10, 2.11). In generalized transduction (Figure 2.10), the infecting phage develops normally, assembling various viral components such as new viral chromosomes, and new "head" and "tail" structures into hundreds of complete phage particles. In doing so, it accidently sequesters genes (in the form of DNA) from its dying host into the "head" structure containing its own intact phage DNA chromosome. After the phage particles are released from the destroyed host cell containing the "accidental" DNA host fragments, they can infect a new (recipient) host cell and release them internally. Of course, under ordinary conditions, the infecting phage would develop normally and destroy the cell. However, there are several circumstances under which it does not develop, permitting the accidental chromosomal fragments from the original cell to integrate its genes into the host chromosome by recombination. This recombination then confers new traits on its host (similar to lysogenic conversion described above). Some of these circumstances involve (1) infecting a cell that is lysogenic (that is, it already has an integrated viral chromosome that inhibits development, but not recombination), and (2) infecting a closely related genus that also inhibits development but not recombination. In specialized transduction (Figure 2.11), a lysogen is somehow activated (or induced by specific chemicals or radiation to produce new phages). In a number of instances, the individual phages can carry a small piece of bacterial DNA that was near the site where the "prophage" was integrated, replacing the phage DNA that had been there before. Although this activated "hybrid" phage can produce new viruses, lyse the host cell, and infect a new strain of bacteria, it cannot develop new phages, but instead it integrates into the bacterial chromosome of the new strain, creating a new lysogenic state. However, the bacterial genes that were also integrated as part of the lysogen can still function to confer new traits on the host as in generalized transduction.

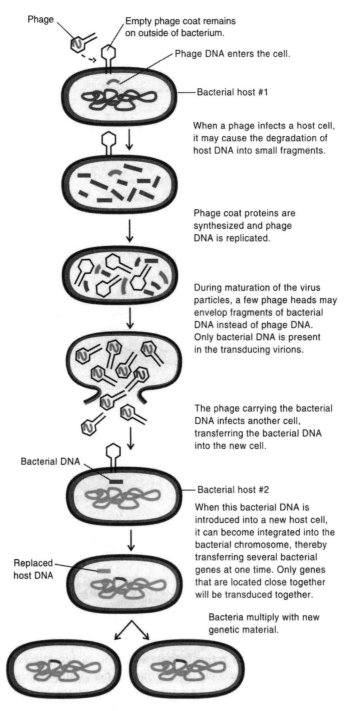

Phage

Empty phage coat remains
on outside of bacterium.

Phage DNA enters the cell.

Bacterial host #1

When a phage infects a host cell,
it may cause the degradation of
host DNA into small fragments.

Phage coat proteins are
synthesized and phage
DNA is replicated.

During maturation of the virus
particles, a few phage heads may
envelop fragments of bacterial
DNA instead of phage DNA.
Only bacterial DNA is present
in the transducing virions.

The phage carrying the bacterial
DNA infects another cell,
transferring the bacterial DNA
into the new cell.

Bacterial DNA

Bacterial host #2

When this bacterial DNA is
introduced into a new host cell,
it can become integrated into the
bacterial chromosome, thereby
transferring several bacterial
genes at one time. Only genes
that are located close together
will be transduced together.

Replaced
host DNA

Bacteria multiply with new
genetic material.

FIGURE 2.10 Transduction (generalized). Any fragment of the chromosomal DNA of the donor cell
can be transferred in this process. All the DNA molecules of the bacterial virus and of the bacteria
are double stranded. (See Plate 12)

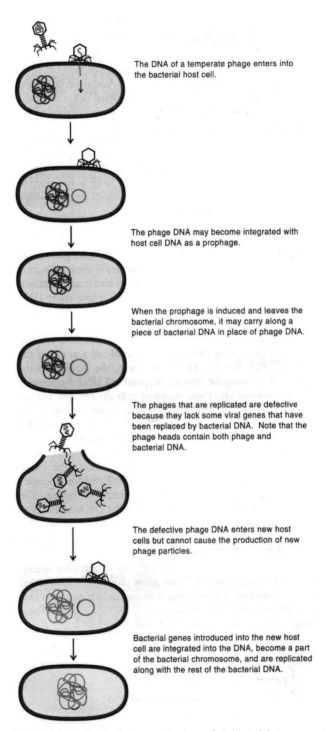

The DNA of a temperate phage enters into the bacterial host cell.

The phage DNA may become integrated with host cell DNA as a prophage.

When the prophage is induced and leaves the bacterial chromosome, it may carry along a piece of bacterial DNA in place of phage DNA.

The phages that are replicated are defective because they lack some viral genes that have been replaced by bacterial DNA. Note that the phage heads contain both phage and bacterial DNA.

The defective phage DNA enters new host cells but cannot cause the production of new phage particles.

Bacterial genes introduced into the new host cell are integrated into the DNA, become a part of the bacterial chromosome, and are replicated along with the rest of the bacterial DNA.

FIGURE 2.11 Specialized transduction by temperate phage. Only bacterial genes near the site where the prophage has integrated can be transduced. (See Plate 13)

An amazing example of how generalized transduction led to the creation of a "new" pathogen was elucidated when bacterial phages that infected and destroyed the pathogen that causes dysentery, *Shigella dysenteriae* (which itself had infected the intestine of its human host), somehow cross-infected a strain of *Escherichia coli*, a common nonpathogenic inhabitant of that same intestine. In doing so, it transduced contaminating *Shigella* genes, which coded for the powerful toxin that causes dysentery (characterized by a severe bloody diarrhea), and these genes became integrated into the *Escherichia coli* chromosome by recombination. This happened a number of years ago. Now we have a new *Escherichia coli* pathogen (O157-H7), which has caused severe outbreaks of dysentery all over the world.

The aforementioned recombination processes (transformation, and viral mediated) are capable of transferring only a limited number of genes to a recipient, not more than about twenty. However, there is one additional major recombination process in bacteria, called "conjugation," where, in fact, almost the entire chromosome can be transferred under the appropriate conditions from a donor cell to a recipient cell (Figure 2.12).

This phenomenon is more analogous to sexual reproduction in higher eukaryotes, because the donor (male) transfers its chromosome to the recipient (female) by intimate contact, using adhesins to attach itself, and then forms a "fertilization" tube through which the donor chromosome is transferred. Integration by recombination with the recipient chromosome soon follows. The entire process is controlled by a small extrachromosomal piece of self-replicating DNA called a plasmid that lives "in harmony" within the (male) bacterial cell. There are many kinds of important plasmids, which will be discussed below, but this particular one, appropriately termed the "fertility" or "F" plasmid, controls which cell acts as the male (the one containing the plasmid) and which is the female (without the plasmid). Interestingly enough, the plasmid can also be transferred to the female, inducing it to become "male." If all this sounds somewhat bizarre, the importance of conjugation lies in its incredible end result; namely, the relatively large interchange of genetic material from two different cells (more than transformation and transduction), which can result in quantum leaps in evolution of the species, or if conjugation occurs between related species, then similar quantum leaps in both.

As if the above genetic-exchange mechanisms weren't enough to provide variability to microorganisms and their pathogens, at least two other phenomena have become of particular importance in transferring virulence genes and genes that enable pathogens to become resistant to antibiotics. The first involves plasmids (defined above), which are ubiquitous throughout the microbial world. One such plasmid group known as "R" or resistance plasmids encodes a variety of genes that either inactivate antibiotics or enable their pathogenic hosts to do so. How and why these plasmid genes arose is obscure, but they can be transferred to other antibiotic-sensitive pathogens,

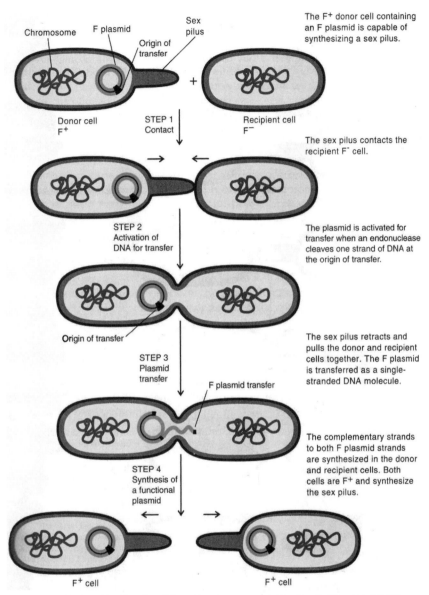

FIGURE 2.12 Conjugation. Transfer of the entire chromosome of the F or fertility plasmid. The exact process by which the donor DNA passes into the recipient cells is not known. (See Plate 14)

even unrelated ones, by conjugation (as indicated above) and can confer antibiotic resistance upon them as well. Such plasmids are called "broad host range" plasmids. Some of the most common antibiotics and other inhibitory drugs that fall prey to this inactivation include streptomycin, tetracyclins, and sulfur drugs. However, other plasmid groups carry genes involved in virulence, such as toxin formation and production of adhesins, which can also be transferred by conjugation. This phenomenon is similar to that of lysogenic conversion (described in a previous section) with bacterial phages that contain such genes, but after infecting their hosts they become integrated into the bacterial chromosome. The end result is the same, rendering a previously harmless bacterial strain highly virulent.

Last but not least are what have been called "jumping genes" or, more accurately, "transposons" (Figure 2.13). These consist of small DNA fragments that exist as part of the bacterial chromosome, often containing genes encoding antibiotic resistance (such as plasmids) but that also encode genetic information "allowing" them to "jump" from one part of the chromosome to another, or even to plasmids. Talk about "weird." Not many geneticists could have visualized such a phenomenon, since the chromosome (or its DNA) was supposed to be very stable and not subject to chaotic moves. Nevertheless, this mechanism can create significant problems for many infected hosts, since, if the transposon moves its antibiotic genes to a broad-host-range plasmid, the latter can then be transferred to other initially nonresistant pathogens by conjugation. Once this occurs, antibiotic resistance genes can become "ubiquitous" throughout many different types of pathogens.

H. Modern Technologies

In recent revolutionary advances of modern genetics, new technologies have been developed (starting in the 1980s) that literally created a firestorm in studying the biology of microorganisms and especially pathogens. Perhaps the most important of these (and the first one developed) is called "genomics," which is defined simply as a determination of the sequence of bases in DNA. Genomics has made it possible to unravel the sequence of every gene contained within the single chromosome (or the entire genotype!) of a number of microorganisms, including deadly pathogens. It is hard to imagine the existence of such technology, when it is recognized that even in a "simple" microorganism such as *Escherichia coli*, there are approximately 4.6 million purine and pyrimidine base pairs. Others range from 1.66 million base pairs in *Helicobacter pylori*, the organism that causes ulcers, to 4.44 million base pairs for the actinomycete that causes tuberculosis. Approximately one thousand bacterial genomes have been sequenced thus far, and new ones are being deciphered almost monthly. What we will focus on briefly is how genomics has aided in the study of bacterial pathogenesis. In a previous section concerning virulence factors, we pointed out that many of the genes are similar regardless of the pathogen, because all pathogens have to accomplish the same tasks to infect the host and to successfully cause the disease. From genomics, it was learned that many of them are located close together on different regions of the chromosome. These regions are called "pathogenicity islands" and are

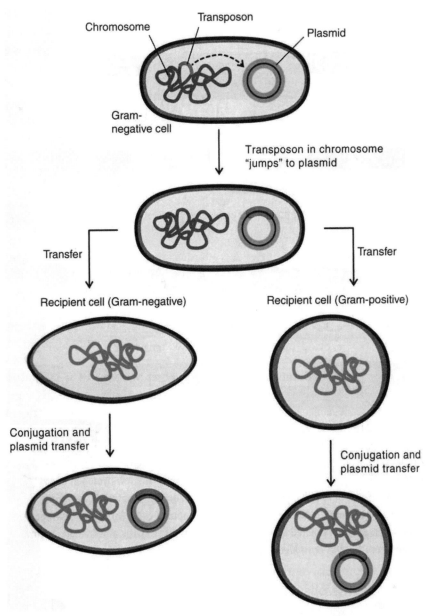

FIGURE 2.13 The movement of a transposon throughout a bacterial population. Note that transfer can be between bacteria belonging to different genera (groups). (See Plate 15)

made up of a number of operons (with regulatory and structural genes) that control their expression. There are other genes on such "islands" for which no role has yet been elucidated, and this is the beauty of the technology. They too may play a hidden role in pathogenesis. Other insights include the fact that nonpathogenic strains do not have these "islands," and that the entire island can be transferred by conjugation to such strains. In another type of study using genomics, the complete sequence of a pathogen that causes upper respiratory infections, *Hemophilus influenzae*, was deciphered in 1995. It produces an endotoxin, that outer-surface complex of lipids, polysaccharides, and protein (LPS for short) responsible for its toxic effects. As one might imagine, there are many genes involved in coding for enzymes that synthesize the various components of the toxin. In twenty years of hard work prior to the era of genomics, approximately twenty-five genes were uncovered by techniques in molecular biology, biochemistry, and genetics. After the advent of genomics, by comparing the genome of *Hemophilus* with other genomes from pathogens that produce endotoxins, as well as nonpathogenic strains, an additional nine genes were revealed within six months. This is not to disparage the previous research, but it just illustrates how powerful a tool genomics is. Of course, the hard work is still to try to elucidate how these new genes function by the techniques just stated and to predict the minimum LPS structure required for an efficient pathogenesis.

There are two additional powerful technologies that have been developed: bioinformatics tries to understand when the myriad of genes revealed by genomics function (or not) in the cell), and, most important, proteomics tries to determine the myriad of proteins that are expressed and how they function. Truly, it is an exciting and important time for revealing how these amazing one-celled creatures do what they do best so quickly and efficiently.

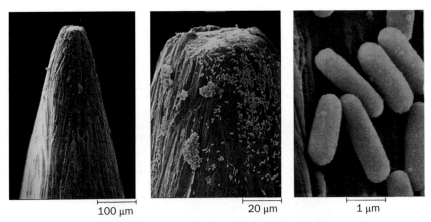

100 µm 20 µm 1 µm

PLATE 1 Bacteria are extremely small. Shown here at various magnifications, cells of the bacterium *Bacillus subtilis* on the tip of a pin. In the scale, µm is a "micrometer" (one millionth of a meter, which is 39.37 inches). (See Figure 1.2)

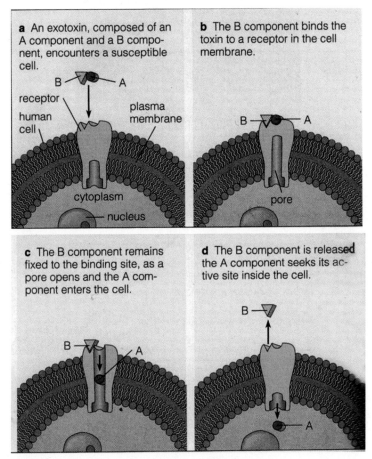

a An exotoxin, composed of an A component and a B component, encounters a susceptible cell.

B — A
receptor
human cell
plasma membrane
cytoplasm
nucleus

b The B component binds the toxin to a receptor in the cell membrane.

B — A
pore

c The B component remains fixed to the binding site, as a pore opens and the A component enters the cell.

B — A

d The B component is released the A component seeks its active site inside the cell.

B —
A

PLATE 2 Exotoxins. The action of some AB toxins. (See Figure 1.4)

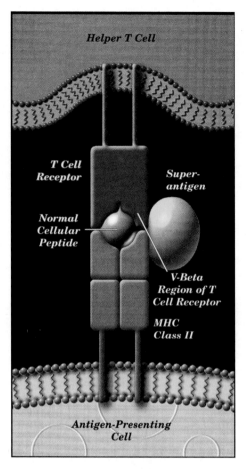

PLATE 3 Superantigens. These exotoxins act to short circuit the specificity of those white blood cells (known as helper "T" lymphocytes and macrophages) that bring the foreign substance (in this case, a fragment of the invading pathogen, known as the antigen) to the attachment site of the "T" lymphocyte, causing them to overproduce inflammatory factors that can damage or destroy host cells. (See Figure 1.5)

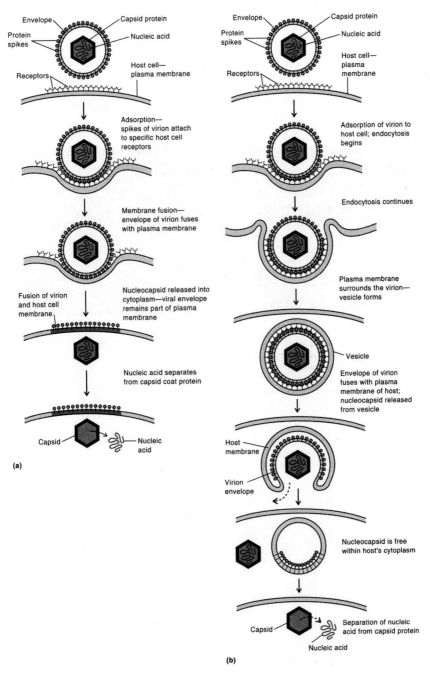

PLATE 4 Entry of enveloped animal viruses into host cells: (a) entry following membrane fusion and (b) entry by endocytosis (a process by which the host cell actually engulfs the virus). (See Figure 1.7)

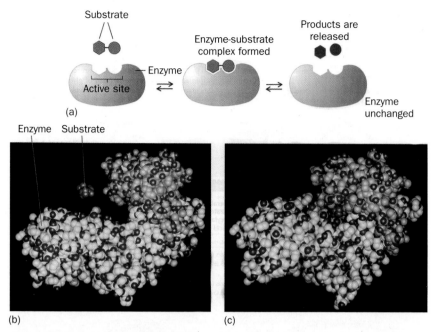

PLATE 5 Mechanism of enzyme action: (a) The substrate binds to the active site, forming an enzyme-substrate complex. The products are then released, leaving the enzyme unchanged and free to combine with new substrate molecules. (b) A model showing an enzyme and its substrate. (c) The binding of the substrate to the active site causes the shape of the flexible enzyme to change slightly. (See Figure 2.2)

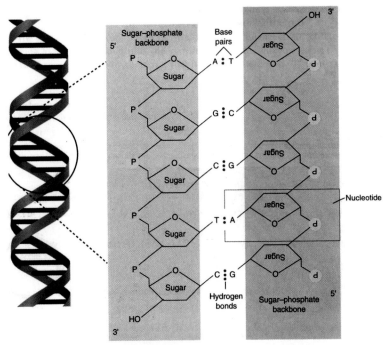

PLATE 6 The double helix of DNA. The two strands of DNA are antiparallel; one strand is oriented to the 5' to 3' direction, and its complement is oriented in the 3' to 5' direction. Hydrogen bonding occurs between the complementary base pairs; three bonds form between a G-C base pair, and two bonds form between an A-T base pair. (See Figure 2.3)

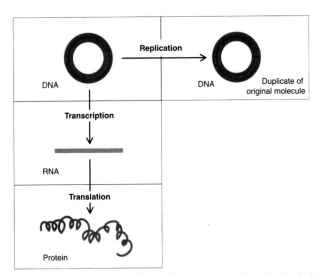

PLATE 7 Overview of replication, transcription, and translation. DNA replication is the process that duplicates DNA, so that its encoded information can be passed on to future generations. Transcription is the process that copies the genetic information into a transitional form, RNA. Translation is the process that deciphers the encoded information to synthesize a specific protein. (See Figure 2.4)

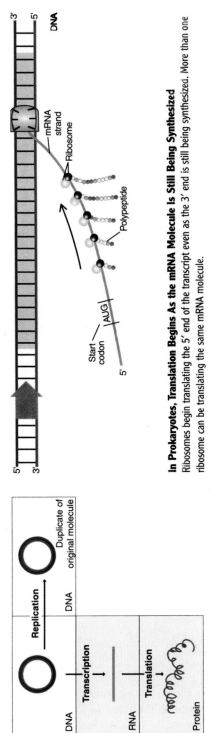

In Prokaryotes, Translation Begins As the mRNA Molecule Is Still Being Synthesized
Ribosomes begin translating the 5' end of the transcript even as the 3' end is still being synthesized. More than one ribosome can be translating the same mRNA molecule.

PLATE 8 In prokaryotes, translation begins as the mRNA molecule is still being synthesized. Ribosomes begin translating the 5' end of the transcript even as the 3' end is still being synthesized. More than one ribosome can be translating the same mRNA molecule. (See Figure 2.5)

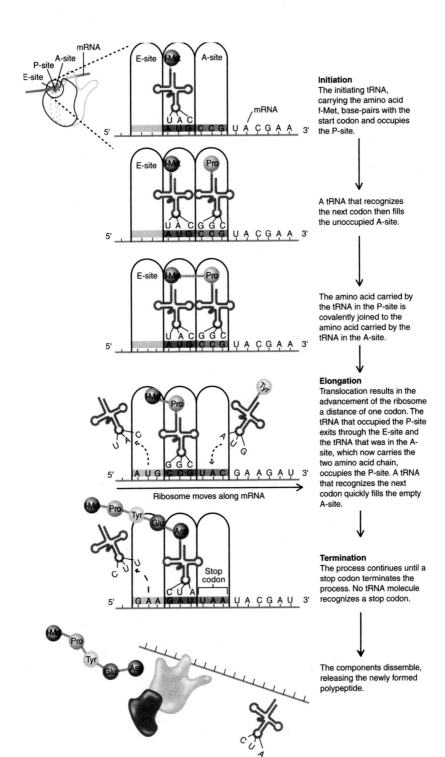

Initiation
The initiating tRNA, carrying the amino acid f-Met, base-pairs with the start codon and occupies the P-site.

A tRNA that recognizes the next codon then fills the unoccupied A-site.

The amino acid carried by the tRNA in the P-site is covalently joined to the amino acid carried by the tRNA in the A-site.

Elongation
Translocation results in the advancement of the ribosome a distance of one codon. The tRNA that occupied the P-site exits through the E-site and the tRNA that was in the A-site, which now carries the two amino acid chain, occupies the P-site. A tRNA that recognizes the next codon quickly fills the empty A-site.

Termination
The process continues until a stop codon terminates the process. No tRNA molecule recognizes a stop codon.

The components dissemble, releasing the newly formed polypeptide.

PLATE 9 The process of translation. (See Figure 2.6)

Mechanism 1

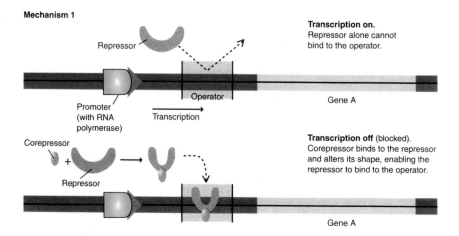

Repressor

Transcription on.
Repressor alone cannot bind to the operator.

Promoter
(with RNA
polymerase)

Operator

Transcription

Gene A

Corepressor

Repressor

Transcription off (blocked).
Corepressor binds to the repressor and alters its shape, enabling the repressor to bind to the operator.

Gene A

Mechanism 2

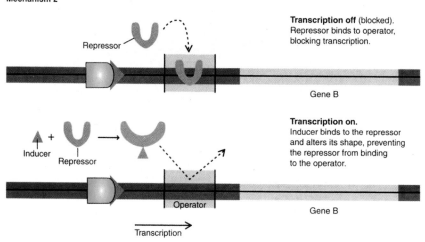

Repressor

Transcription off (blocked).
Repressor binds to operator, blocking transcription.

Gene B

Inducer

Repressor

Transcription on.
Inducer binds to the repressor and alters its shape, preventing the repressor from binding to the operator.

Operator

Gene B

Transcription

PLATE 10 Transcriptional regulation by repressors (the operon). (See Figure 2.7)

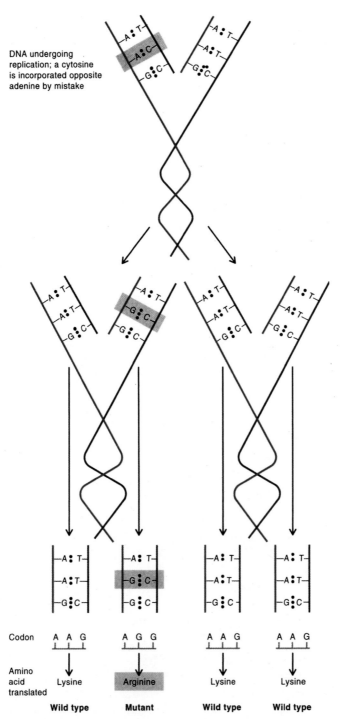

DNA undergoing replication; a cytosine is incorporated opposite adenine by mistake

PLATE 11 Base substitution. Shown here is the generation of a mutant organism as a result of the incorporation of a pyrimidine base (cytosine) in place of thymine in DNA replication. (See Figure 2.9)

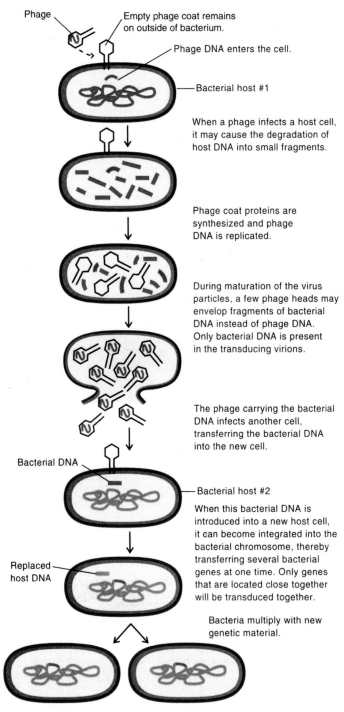

Phage

Empty phage coat remains on outside of bacterium.

Phage DNA enters the cell.

Bacterial host #1

When a phage infects a host cell, it may cause the degradation of host DNA into small fragments.

Phage coat proteins are synthesized and phage DNA is replicated.

During maturation of the virus particles, a few phage heads may envelop fragments of bacterial DNA instead of phage DNA. Only bacterial DNA is present in the transducing virions.

The phage carrying the bacterial DNA infects another cell, transferring the bacterial DNA into the new cell.

Bacterial DNA

Bacterial host #2

When this bacterial DNA is introduced into a new host cell, it can become integrated into the bacterial chromosome, thereby transferring several bacterial genes at one time. Only genes that are located close together will be transduced together.

Replaced host DNA

Bacteria multiply with new genetic material.

PLATE 12 Transduction (generalized). Any fragment of the chromosomal DNA of the donor cell can be transferred in this process. All the DNA molecules of the bacterial virus and of the bacteria are double stranded. (See Figure 2.10)

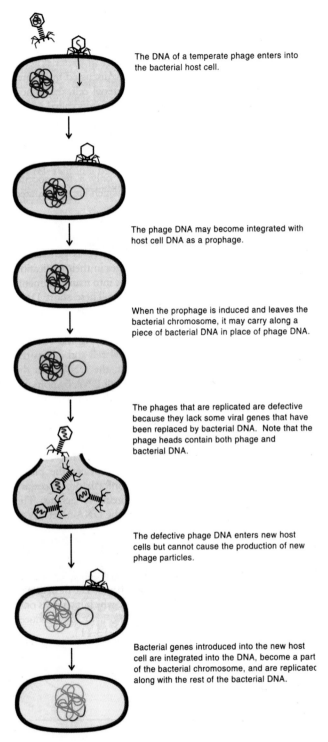

The DNA of a temperate phage enters into the bacterial host cell.

The phage DNA may become integrated with host cell DNA as a prophage.

When the prophage is induced and leaves the bacterial chromosome, it may carry along a piece of bacterial DNA in place of phage DNA.

The phages that are replicated are defective because they lack some viral genes that have been replaced by bacterial DNA. Note that the phage heads contain both phage and bacterial DNA.

The defective phage DNA enters new host cells but cannot cause the production of new phage particles.

Bacterial genes introduced into the new host cell are integrated into the DNA, become a part of the bacterial chromosome, and are replicated along with the rest of the bacterial DNA.

PLATE 13 Specialized transduction by temperate phage. Only bacterial genes near the site where the prophage has integrated can be transduced. (See Figure 2.11)

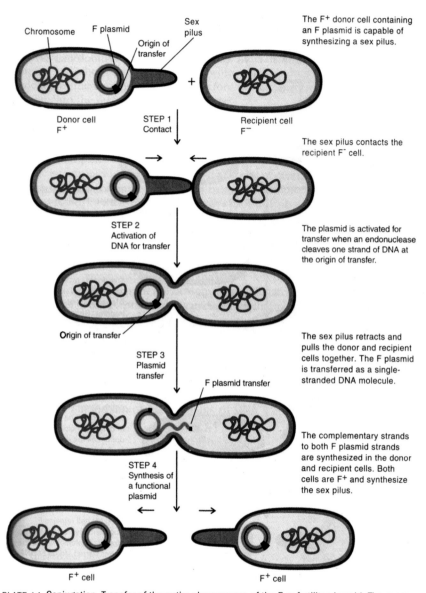

PLATE 14 Conjugation. Transfer of the entire chromosome of the F or fertility plasmid. The exact process by which the donor DNA passes into the recipient cells is not known. (See Figure 2.12)

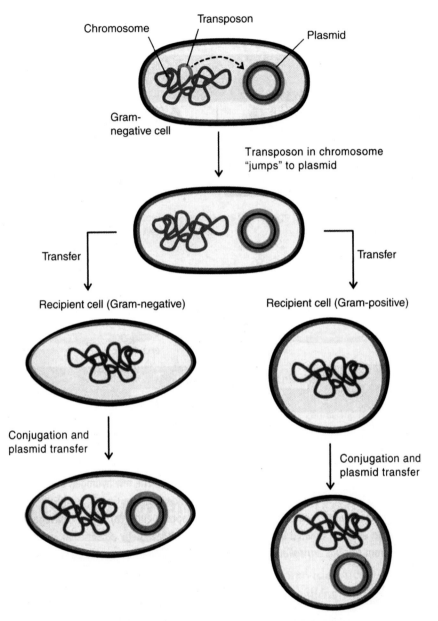

PLATE 15 The movement of a transposon throughout a bacterial population. Note that transfer can be between bacteria belonging to different genera (groups). (See Figure 2.13)

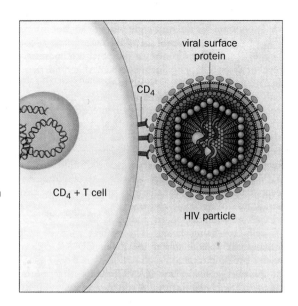

PLATE 16 Infection by HIV. Sketch of how viral surface proteins attach to CD4 receptors in the first step of infection. A CD4 $^+$ T cell is a lymphocyte, a type of white blood cell involved in managing the production of antibodies. (See Figure 5.1)

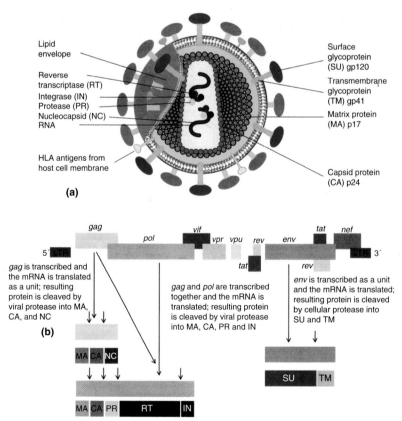

PLATE 17 Human immunodeficiency virus, type 1 (HIV-1). (a) Diagrammatic representation of the virus, showing important protein antigens. (b) Map of the HIV-1 genome, showing its nine genes and flanking long-terminal repeats (LTRs). The LTRs contain regulatory sequences recognized by the host cell. (c) HIV-1 gene products. The accessory gene products are translated into proteins of final size, while *gag* and *pol* products must be cleaved by viral protease, and *env* products by host cell protease. The small arrows indicate the sites of cleavage. (See Figure 5.2)

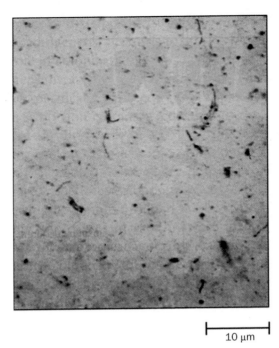

10 μm

PLATE 18 *Mycobacterium tuberculosis* as seen in sputum from an individual with tuberculosis. The sputum has been "digested," meaning it has been treated with strong alkali to kill the other bacteria that are invariably present. (See Figure 5.3)

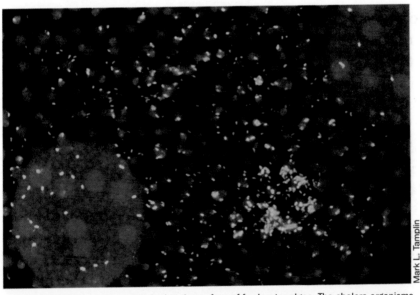

Mark L. Tamplin

PLATE 19 Cholera organisms attached to the surface of freshwater algae. The cholera organisms are stained green. The red color is due to the fluorescence of chlorophyll A in the algae. (See Figure 5.11)

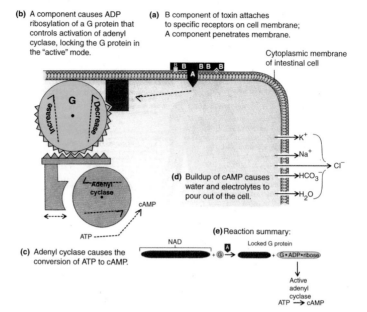

(b) A component causes ADP ribosylation of a G protein that controls activation of adenyl cyclase, locking the G protein in the "active" mode.

(a) B component of toxin attaches to specific receptors on cell membrane; A component penetrates membrane.

Cytoplasmic membrane of intestinal cell

Increase / Decrease

G

Adenyl cyclase

ATP

cAMP

(d) Buildup of cAMP causes water and electrolytes to pour out of the cell.

K^+
Na^+
Cl^-
HCO_3^-
H_2O

(c) Adenyl cyclase causes the conversion of ATP to cAMP.

(e) Reaction summary:

NAD

A

Locked G protein

$G \cdot ADP \cdot ribose$

Active adenyl cyclase
ATP → cAMP

Mode of Action of Cholera Toxin As with other A-B toxins, the B portion attaches the toxin to the host cell, and the A portion penetrates the cell and causes toxicity. In this case, the target of the A portion is a G protein responsible for regulating productoin of cAMP.

PLATE 20 How cholera exotoxin acts on the cell. (See Figure 5.12)

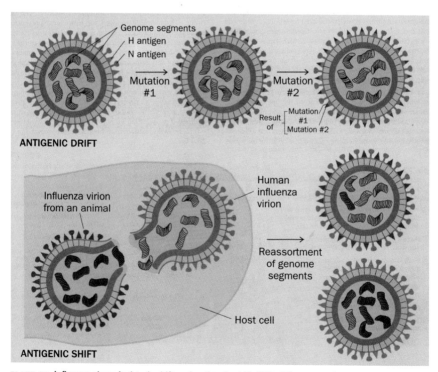

Genome segments
H antigen
N antigen

Mutation #1

Mutation #2

Result of Mutation #1, Mutation #2

ANTIGENIC DRIFT

Influenza virion from an animal

Human influenza virion

Reassortment of genome segments

Host cell

ANTIGENIC SHIFT

PLATE 21 Influenza virus: Antigenic drift and antigenic shift. With drift, repeated mutations cause gradual change in the antigens composing the hemagglutinin, so that antibody against the original virus becomes progressively less effective. With shift, there is an abrupt, major change in the hemagglutinin antigens because the virus acquires a new genome segment, which in this case codes for hemagglutinin. Changes in neuraminidase could occur by the same mechanism. (See Figure 5.13)

3

History of Microbiology

It is appropriate to briefly discuss microbiology in a historical perspective because so much of it was based on a search for the causes of infectious diseases. If one could divide up the various "ages" of microbiology, three of them would be recognized, which are "quaintly" described as (1) Voices in the Wilderness, (2) the Golden Age, and (3) the Modern Era.

A. Voices in the Wilderness

One could go as far back as antiquity for the first age where a number of important activities of microorganisms were recognized but not understood, except as metaphysical processes (or a philosophical analysis of the ultimate causes of nature, as defined by the great Aristotle himself). These included fermentation, decay, and the causes of disease. Indeed, this view was not unreasonable at the time, since microorganisms were so small that they were invisible to the naked eye. Their very discovery depended on the development of an optical science, which was nonexistent then. Yet, there were a few "voices in the wilderness" such as the Italian monk Fracastorius, who in 1546 suggested that a "contagum vivum" (literally, bad air) was responsible for the spread of disease (which was why aristocrats quickly retired to their country estates to avoid contact with the "peasants" during the many plagues that constantly beset the crowded towns and villages). Others, such as the German "scientist" Plenciz (1762), also asserted that diseases are caused by minute organisms floating in the air. However, it remained for the first "father" of microbiology, the Dutchman Anton van Leeuwenhoek, who was the most skillful lens grinder of his time, to visualize these "invisible" microorganisms in the late 1600s. Using only simple lenses in a simple light microscope that he constructed, he examined many natural "environments" and saw not only bacteria, but also algae, protozoa, sperm cells, and red blood cells. His drawings of bacterial shape and motility are accurate even by today's standards. Yet, due to the lack of similar instruments, other scientists doubted van Leeuwenhoek's discoveries until better (compound) microscopes were developed nearly a century later. Then several other voices were heard. The first was the Danish zoologist O. Muller, who in 1786 revealed structural details within bacteria not observed previously, by using the more advanced microscopes. The second was the German scientist Ehrenberg, who in 1838 was the first to separate different groups of microorganisms by culturing them in enriched nutrient solutions. In effect, this was the first classification of microorganisms. However, it remained for the English doctor E. Jenner (Figure 3.1) in 1796 to perform the first "vaccination" (as we call it now) of individuals to protect them from the dreaded disease smallpox. He removed some fluid from a lesion of a "milkmaid" who had a related but not as deadly a disease as smallpox, called cowpox, which could be transmitted from cows to humans (a typical zoonoses).

He then "inoculated" (injected) a healthy boy with the material, who promptly developed cowpox. Next, Jenner did something that today would be so ethically monstrous that he would be put away for years; namely, inoculate the boy with material from a smallpox lesion. Nothing happened! In other words, the boy developed immunity to cowpox, which was close enough (as a virus) to smallpox so that he also became immune to the latter. Of course, Jenner knew nothing about viruses, but he had the insight to use principles of

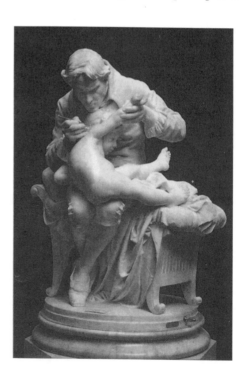

FIGURE 3.1 A statue of Edward Jenner vaccinating a child against smallpox.

vaccination that are used even today—namely, the use of a "weak" (or attenuated) form of a pathogen as a vaccine in order to induce resistance against the more virulent form.

B. The Golden Age and Modern Era

So ends the first age of "voices in the wilderness." The second era, which is referred to as the "golden age," started in the middle 1880s with remarkable advances in elucidating the "germ theory of disease." Two giants of microbiology were initially responsible for this age: one French, Louis Pasteur, and one German, Robert Koch (Figures 3.2, 3.3).

Pasteur (Figure 3.2) was a chemist by training and first became interested in the "diseases" of beer and wine that occurred when the fermentation process resulted in the production of vinegar instead of alcohol. It had previously been thought that the shift to vinegar was due to processes carried out by

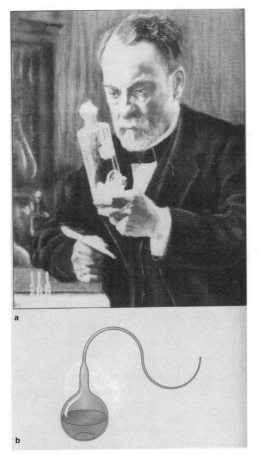

a

b

FIGURE 3.2 (a) Louis Pasteur in his laboratory. (b) In 1861 he devised this swan-necked flask to prove that microorganisms did not generate spontaneously in sterilized broth exposed to air.

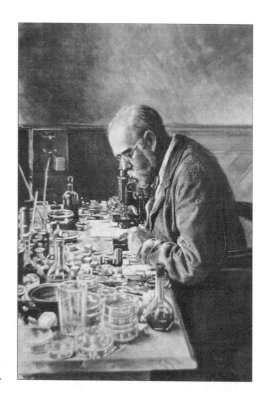

FIGURE 3.3 Robert Koch, another
giant in microbiology, in his laboratory.

dying bacteria, which he demonstrated were in fact due to living ones. To treat
this condition, Pasteur in 1864 invented the process of "pasteurization" (mild
heating of the wine for a short period of time at a temperature of 70°C, which
would kill most of the bacteria, followed by cooling) to render it much less
likely to produce vinegar. Thus, this process, which has since been employed
for almost two centuries in the processing of raw milk and other drinkable
fluids consumed by humans, has saved countless individuals from becoming
infected by diseases such as tuberculosis and food poisoning. However, that
is only a small sample of what Pasteur accomplished. Delving deeper into the
nature of microbes and their effects on humans, he proposed the first germ
theory of disease after studying particular infectious diseases such as anthrax
and tuberculosis; his theory stated that "microorganisms were solely responsible for the pathological conditions of the particular disease." Although we take
this concept for granted today, it was a revolutionary concept then. Pasteur
also confirmed Jenner's vaccination model with two deadly diseases, rabies
and anthrax. Using ingenious methods for creating attenuated forms of pathogens (virus in the case of rabies, and bacteria in the case of anthrax), he cured
a number of rabies victims who had already been bitten by "mad" dogs, which
was amazing since they had exhibited early signs of the fatal disease. Apparently, his weakened vaccine (which came from monkeys) stimulated massive

amounts of antibodies that also inactivated the stronger form. Robert Koch, a German physician (Figure 3.3), not only studied dreaded diseases such as tuberculosis and cholera but developed the experimental methods necessary for the proof of the germ theory of disease. In 1876, he published his four "postulates" for relating a specific microorganism to a specific disease (Figure 3.4).

Now known as "Koch's postulates," they serve us even today for this purpose. First, an organism should be present in hosts suffering from the disease, but not in healthy ones. Second, the organism should be isolated from its sick host and cultured in suitable nutrient solutions. Third, inoculation (or introduction) of the organism into a healthy host should produce the characteristic disease (of course, this is not performed on humans, but rather in experimental animals, which could be a problem if only humans can be infected). And fourth, the organism should be reisolated from the diseased animal and verified that it is identical to the original isolate. However, what Koch should really be remembered for is that he devised a nutrient culture, which enabled microbiologists to isolate a suspected pathogen in "pure" form. Up until Koch's time, it was impossible to purify a particular isolate from an infected host because there was no way to separate it from contaminating microorganisms. One could use techniques to "enrich" the organism only in a particular nutrient environment. Koch simply added a solidifying agent (gelatin, a protein that can be heated in solution to dissolve it, which then hardens at lower temperatures) to hot liquid nutrient solutions and then allowed it to solidify at room temperature. When an isolate (with other contaminants) was spread on such a hardened nutrient medium (as it is called), discrete visible "colonies" were observed after a short growth period. Since these colonies were of all different shapes (but usually round) and sizes, Koch realized that they were the result of different individual microorganisms that had been trapped in the solid medium and grew in place where they were deposited. Thus, each colony could contain millions of individual bacterial cells, all descendent from the original one deposited on the surface of the solid medium. Not only did Koch use this knowledge to study specific pathogens, but the technique led to the discovery of new pathogens by many microbiologists all over the world. We cannot list them all, but the following represents some of the more important ones.

Klebs, 1883, diphtheria
Frankel, 1886, pneumonia
Wechselbaum, 1887, meningitis
Kitasato, 1889, tetanus
Yersin, 1894, bubonic plague
Francis, 1904, tularemia (rabbit fever)
Bang, 1905, brucellosis (undulant fever)

There were numerous other momentous discoveries during the golden age that related to many other aspects of pathogenicity, such as the discovery of

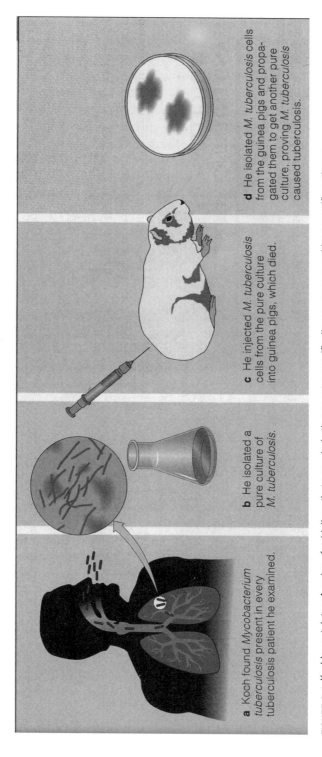

a Koch found *Mycobacterium tuberculosis* present in every tuberculosis patient he examined.

b He isolated a pure culture of *M. tuberculosis*.

c He injected *M. tuberculosis* cells from the pure culture into guinea pigs, which died.

d He isolated *M. tuberculosis* cells from the guinea pigs and propagated them to get another pure culture, proving *M. tuberculosis* caused tuberculosis.

FIGURE 3.4 Koch's postulates: A series of guidelines that proved whether or not a specific disease was caused by a specific pathogen.

viruses in 1898 by Iwanowski and Beijerinck, the first use of chemicals to treat diseases by P. Ehrlich in 1908 (his so-called magic bullet, which was used to successfully treat syphilis patients), and the discovery by P. Rous in 1913 that certain viruses can cause cancer in chickens. Suffice it to say, all of them led to the "modern era," which would encompass a telephone book of a large city were we to list all the names and their significant discoveries. Of course, our previous discussions have, in fact, discussed a number of those discoveries related to microbes, their activities, and their pathogenicity.

4

Emerging and Reemerging Diseases

A. Introduction

It is astounding, really, that in almost every newspaper, every day, it is probable that an article or account will appear concerning an outbreak of a specific infectious disease somewhere on our planet (Figure 4.1). Whether it concerns well-known maladies such as whooping cough or pneumonia, or new ones such as EBOLA or SARS, their effects on our psyches are profound. There are feelings of unease, fear, and surprise that such outbreaks either should occur at all, because of well-known ways to treat them, or have not been recognized previously.

Yet, these perceptions could be ameliorated if the many factors involved in the outbreaks were more clearly understood. Of course, in some cases of a completely new disease, such factors are unknown, although with time, most of them fall to the relentless onslaught of modern research, which was not always the case in years past. For example, the sudden appearance of SARS (severe acute respiratory syndrome) in China, which caused a brief but deadly havoc in 2003, also galvanized a huge international effort coordinated by the World Health Organization to find its cause (a new "corona" virus) and how to contain it (by stringent methods of quarantine). In less than four months, the outbreaks were controlled by public and private health workers who cared for the infected patients. Amazingly enough, SARS has apparently disappeared (genetic variation?), although a vaccine has been developed that may not be tested despite the fact that the disease could reemerge. For a variety of other infectious diseases, however, which either should not have occurred or should have been contained, the factors involved in their reappearance are troubling. For example, tuberculosis is still the world's leading killer of adults and has reemerged strongly in such cities as New York, London, and Tokyo, due, in part, to the continued rise in AIDS cases, which affect the hosts' immune system,

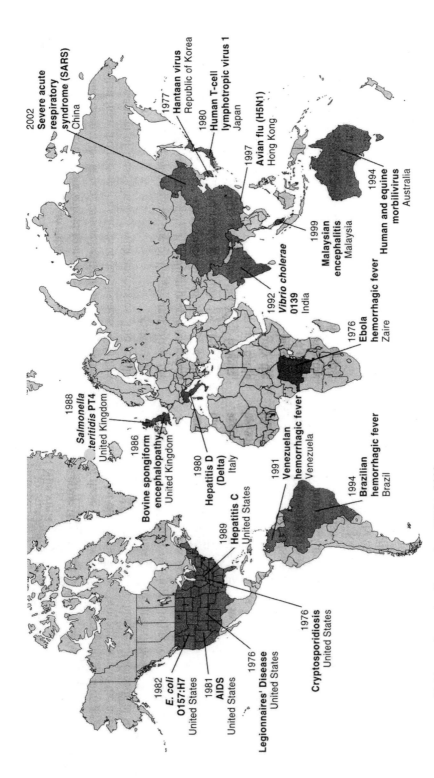

FIGURE 4.1 World map of emerging diseases from 1976 to 2002.

allowing previously dormant organisms to multiply. In addition, resistance to multiple antibiotics has also played a role in a continued increase of the disease. Particularly startling are outbreaks of disease such as diphtheria (in the former Soviet Union) and whooping cough (in the United States), for which effective vaccines have been available for many years. Apparently, there have been lax enforcement policies where health officials do not require a vaccination of children or do not distribute the vaccine. It is possible to argue that there are many underlying causes for these diseases, which are difficult if not impossible to control; these causes include poverty, poor nutrition, poor housing, and poor sanitary conditions, especially in what we euphemistically call the Third World or the developing world. Nevertheless, if these causes can be defined more rigorously, they can lead to better methods for education, detection, and action.

B. Definitions

So, let us define our terms. Emerging diseases are infectious outbreaks that suddenly erupt in a specific population, or that are rapidly increasing in numbers and geographical range in a population, or that appear in a new host population. These outbreaks can be due to well-known pathogens or to completely new ones. By far, the most common factor in inducing the outbreak is human activities, which then are influenced by direct and indirect "societal" mechanisms, of which three outstanding patterns can be identified. As discussed in a comprehensive lecture presented some years ago at the national meeting of the American Society for Microbiology by an eminent epidemiologist, Neal Nathanson, they include rapid transportation, an explosive increase in the human population, and catastrophic upsets of the environment, either natural or man made. Starting with the first, over the last one hundred years, the speed and availability of transportation has increased remarkably along with massive increases in people who use such transportation worldwide. Thus, it is now possible for someone to be infected with a pathogen at one location and, before symptoms appear, to travel to another location and spread that infection to other individuals, depending on the pathogen. For the second pattern, human populations continue to increase geometrically, with an increasing proportion of the total living in "megacities" (such as, for example, the Washington to Boston axis on the East Coast of the United States, with a population of twenty-five to thirty million people). This inevitable overcrowding favors the more rapid spread of infectious diseases. Finally, third, in many parts of the world there have been major disruptions in the environment, ranging from dam building (such as the Aswan Dam on the Nile River in Egypt, which allowed brackish water to propagate many types of parasites), to deforestation of previously untouched regions such as the Amazon rain forest or jungles in Africa, which caused exposure to hitherto obscure pathogens such as EBOLA and HIV (AIDS) because of road building to access remote areas, and lastly, to massive movement and resettlement of refugees from war-torn countries in Europe, Asia, and Africa. Not only have these three patterns accelerated exposure of humans to new and existing infectious agents, but they also have increased the possibility of new diseases of animals and plants, which then could affect crops and food animals. It should also be noted that attempts to treat these "obscure" diseases (especially AIDS) by injection of new drugs has resulted in further spread of the disease through the increase use of contaminated syringes and needles.

How have these societal factors resulted in an emerging or reemerging infectious disease? There are several mechanisms involved. They include (1) recognition of a previously unidentified entity (most of these in the last thirty years have involved deadly viruses such as the EBOLA, Lassa, and Marburg agents in Africa), (2) the sudden increase in severe illness of a population already infected with an agent that initially results in only a minor illness (such as the virus that causes polio), (3) reemergence of well-known diseases either because of a failure in public health vaccinations, or overuse of antibiotics that causes resistance (examples include bacterial and viral agents such as tuberculosis, cholera, diphtheria, whooping cough, pneumonia, polio, influenza, and measles), (4) new diseases caused by well-known agents that either were completely benign (nonpathogenic) or did cause another mild or severe infection, (5) recognition that a new disease thought to be caused by one pathogen was, in fact, caused by another, and (6) new diseases that result from invasion of a new host population, such as the zoonoses (crossing species barriers to infect humans) described in a previous section. Two of the more "famous" examples include HIV (causing AIDS) and mad cow disease. Although some of the "distinctions" listed above may appear subtle, they do account for most of the outbreaks observed in the recent past.

C. Examples of Each

Although we cannot discuss examples from all five categories in detail, it is instructive to at least illustrate the many "twists and turns" that were manifested for several of the outbreaks, including unexpected ones. In many ways it is very similar to solving a crime: part luck, part insight, and, above all, requiring time and patience. The first example (characteristic of "2" above) is that of polio (or poliomyelitis) (Figure 4.2). This "enterovirus" disease first appeared as an epidemic in Sweden and the United States at the beginning of the twentieth century and continued well into the 1950s, until the famous Salk vaccine was developed in 1955.

It was a dreaded disease of the central nervous system, affecting mostly children and causing paralysis (commonly known as infantile paralysis), requiring

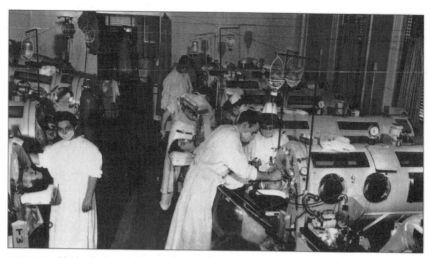

FIGURE 4.2 Mechanical respirators, called iron lungs, were used to keep patients alive during the polio epidemics of the 1940s and 1950s.

them to be placed into an "iron lung" to facilitate breathing. Yet, for many years it was known to be a relatively "harmless" viral ailment that infected most humans at a very early age, with a strong immunity either being induced by the individual or being already present, the immunity being transmitted by a nursing mother through her breast milk. In addition, infections were spread very easily in dense populations, such as in cities, and in common public recreation areas such as beaches. In a very small number of cases, the virus could accidentally invade the spinal cord to cause the disease. So what happened? Incredibly enough, advances in sanitation and personal hygiene, coupled with a greater desire not to expose children to "overcrowded" conditions as well as a greater percentage of mothers who were advised that nursing was unnecessary, seemed to be the culprits. With more children isolated from their peers, and with improved sanitation and less nursing, many of them were not exposed to the virus for quite some time, until they were teenagers or young adults. Thus, when they inevitably were infected (such as in school or by engaging in more social activities), they had no immunity, resulting in a greater possibility for accidental invasion of the spinal cord. One famous example is that of our thirty-second president, Franklin D. Roosevelt, who contracted polio as a young adult, perhaps because his lifestyle was one of wealth and privilege.

The second example (characteristic of "5" above) is that of "mad cow" disease or its scientific name, bovine spongiform encephalopathy (BSE) (Figure 4.3). Of all the bizarre twists and turns for an emerging disease, this one is most unusual in its complex causes.

It all started in 1973, when one of the several Arab-Israeli wars broke out (this one begun by Egypt), which led to the Arab oil boycott of Western

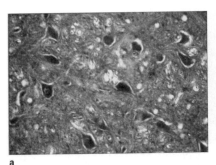 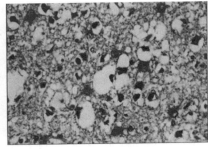

a   b

FIGURE 4.3 Comparison of normal brain tissue (a) and the spongiform brain tissue (b) taken from a patient with Creutzfeldt-Jakob disease.

nations. Not only was gasoline in short supply, but many products derived from petroleum-like solvents were also hard to obtain. As a result, the manner in which animal feed for dairy herds and cattle was prepared was altered, particularly in England. Such food was mostly in the form of protein supplements (called offal), which were derived from slaughtered sheep that were usually treated with petroleum solvents to clean or extract the offal. When a non-petroleum substitute was used, certain "infectious" proteins that are now known as "prions" (see below), which were very common in sheep (causing a deadly neurological disease called scrapie) and had been inactivated by petroleum solvents, "escaped" chemical degradation and were "eaten" by cattle. This practice continued for some time or up until the first appearance of BSE in 1985 in these animals as a new neurological disease. Most of you probably have seen the pitiful videos of "mad" cows, stumbling around enclosures, hardly able to stand. The symptoms were very similar to sheep scrapie, which led investigators to suspect some kind of transmission from sheep through the offal. Although we cannot discuss the nature of prions in great detail, they are not viruses but instead are proteins (of which there are a number of different types) that do not form in the right way in the body. They are known to be responsible for at least a half dozen neurodegenerative diseases in animals and humans, which are always fatal but require a long time to develop. Insidiously enough, they induce normal forms of the protein (for which we still do not know its function) also to form abnormally. All the diseases are characterized by destruction of nerve cells (neurons) in the brain, and the brain itself develops "spongelike" holes. The height of mad cow disease lasted until the mid-1990s, when long after the Arab boycott had ended, new types of food supplements were used that were not derived from sheep. Probably, interest in the disease would have ended if not for a new chapter in the mad cow saga that began in 1996. Ten cases of a neurodegenerative disease appeared in young English adults, which was similar to an inherited disease that occurred only in older people, called Creutzfeldt-Jakob disease (CJD), and which was caused by prions. It was suspected that these new cases (now called "variant" or VCJD) could have been due to eating "prion"-infected meat, which was difficult to prove, but unfortunately the possibility did lead to huge political problems for the English government, whose meat products were banned all over the world. In 2004, definitive studies removed all doubts that, in fact, VCJD is related to mad cow disease. Scottish researchers discovered that the type (or species) of prion present in mad cows is exactly the same (called the BSE signature) as that recovered from autopsies of young adults who had died of VCJD. Although thus far only twenty-one people in England have developed VCJD (and none in the United States), the fear of mad cow disease spreading is always palpable and is highlighted in the media.

The third and last example (characteristic of "4" above) is that of scarlet fever (Figure 4.4). We have previously discussed this well-known disease (caused by a streptococcus bacterium known as *Streptococcus pyogenes*), which seems to have "moderated" from one hundred years ago when it was a deadly disease, producing fatalities as high as 30%, especially in young children, by expressing a strong toxin, among other virulence factors.

However, today, it rarely occurs, with its primary vestige being the common "strep sore throat." Where did it go? It is believed that selective evolutionary pressures (natural selection) played a decisive role to ameliorate the infection precisely because of the societal factors described at the beginning of this section. The spread of this pathogen worldwide (a pandemic) eventually resulted in its demise as it passed through millions and millions of diverse individuals, reaching equilibrium to enhance the survival of both. However, was

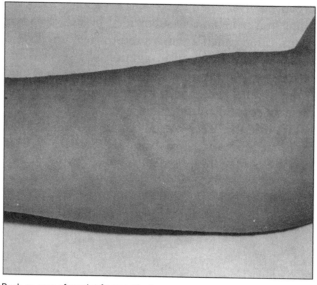

FIGURE 4.4 Rash on arm of scarlet fever patient.

that the "end of the story"? No way! As discussed in a highly informative lecture several years ago by Richard Kraus, former director of the National Institute of Allergy and Infectious Diseases, there are tantalizing clues that genetic information to express the scarlet fever toxin "jumped" from this particular streptococcus to another related one to cause streptococcal toxic shock syndrome (STSS) (see Figure 2.13 for how this could occur). This newly emerging disease has become more frequent and more deadly in many parts of the world and has been hyped by the media as the "flesh-eating disease" that can "kill" in hours. Usually begun as a local skin infection from a minor wound, it rapidly produces an extensive lesion that destroys skin tissue rapidly and is often followed by organ failure, toxic shock, and death. Antibiotics cannot prevent the rapid sequence of events that occur, and patients' lives can be saved in severe cases only by amputation of the infected limbs. By the use of modern molecular genetic and biochemical techniques (genomics and bioinformatics), it was demonstrated that the genes for toxin production, and other genetic "markers" in the STSS-causing streptococcus, correlate strongly with the genes that express scarlet fever toxin of *Streptococcus pyogenes*. Whether it is exactly the same as the disease that killed those victims one hundred years ago must wait further refined analysis by genomics from preserved tissues. Nevertheless, it is an amazing example of possible horizontal gene transfer and how evolution can play deadly "tricks" on our ability to cope with emerging pathogens.

D. Role of Antibiotics

A particularly important factor involved in explaining why infectious diseases that were treated successfully in the past with antimicrobial agents have re-emerged with a vengeance is antibiotic resistance. Unfortunately, perhaps, such resistance is unavoidable because it encompasses the inexorable march of bacterial evolution, which is impossible to stop. As discussed briefly previously, antibiotics, which are chemical compounds produced by living microorganisms that destroy or inhibit the growth of other microorganisms (Figures 4.5 and 4.6) and which have been the mainstay of our treatment of many infectious diseases, have become less and less effective over time. Either by mutations in specific genes whose products are targeted by antibiotics, or by horizontal gene transfer of resistance genes by plasmids and transposons, pathogens have "learned" to overcome them, even when multiple antibiotics are used. Unfortunately, the fear of multiple resistance and "superbugs" (which resist all antibiotics) has been played up mercilessly and unnecessarily by the media for ratings. Not that such resistance shouldn't be a concern, but, in fact, there is no pathogen that eventually cannot be overcome by proper treatment; if not by antibiotics, then by other drugs or vaccines. Moreover, the media rarely emphasize that the infections are almost never fatal, except under

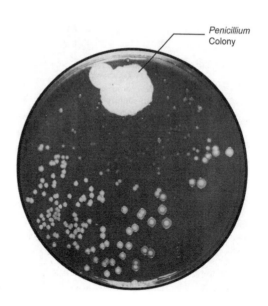

Penicillium
Colony

FIGURE 4.5 This is the actual petri dish that led to the discovery of penicillin in 1929. The plate on which the disease-causing bacterium *Staphylococcus aureus* was being cultivated accidentally became contaminated by a fungal spore that developed into a colony of *Penicillium*. By producing penicillin, the fungus killed or damaged colonies closest to it.

certain circumstances such as lack of any health care. Antibiotics still are of great utility in treatment of many bacterial infectious diseases.

There are ways in which such resistance can be reversible, albeit gradually, of which the most important (at least in our industrialized world) is the cessation of the indiscriminate use of antibiotics. Their overuse by physicians for

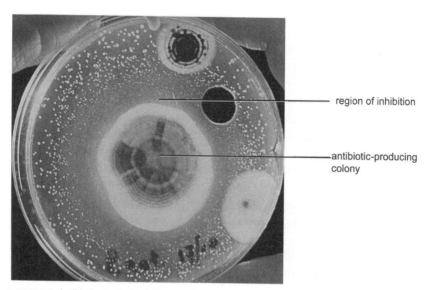

region of inhibition

antibiotic-producing colony

FIGURE 4.6 Antibiotic-producing microorganisms. A plate inoculated with soil often has colonies, such as the larger one in the center of the plate (with brown, spore-covered center and colorless, spore-free edge). Note how the small, white colonies become smaller the closer they are to the antibiotic-producing colony.

ailments such as colds (supposedly to prevent secondary infections)—which are unaffected because they are caused by viruses, their use by legitimate patients who fail to complete their course of antibiotic treatment, their inclusion in animal feed, and their incorporation into everything from mouthwashes to shampoo has accelerated the rise of resistant pathogens. Fortunately, this is not a big problem in the Third World, primarily because such miracle drugs are unavailable and cost too much. As a result, infectious agents have not been exposed to their lethal effects. That is the conundrum: how to balance the needs of the "have nots" with those of the "haves." It is axiomatic that in the former, there is hardly an infectious disease that could not be treated successfully with antibiotics, whereas in the latter, resistance to many of them exceeds 50%, especially in hospitals. It might be thought that pharmaceutical firms that pioneered the search for antibiotics would be encouraged to seek new ones.

In fact, the experience has been the opposite. The number of new antibiotics has been on the decline in recent years because of financial and social considerations. For example, there is a highly competitive market filled with antibiotics that are relatively cheap to produce and target only a limited clientele (but only in the industrialized world). Also, doctors and public health officials do not wish to use new antibiotics except as a last resort for resistant pathogens. And so it goes.

Let us now, however, discuss a number of aspects of antibiotics on a scientific level. Most antibiotics function by inhibiting various stages of protein and nucleic-acid synthesis in bacteria, either by inactivating specific enzymes involved in their syntheses or by binding to specific components such as DNA or RNA to inhibit their functions in replication or transcription. They can also bind to the cell surface of the pathogen and "punch" holes in it. Usually there are two outcomes for the pathogen when they are exposed to a successful antibiotic, which are termed bactericidal or bacteriostatic. The former outcome results in a complete destruction (lysis) of the bacterial cell by several mechanisms, including what is called "self suicide," whereas the latter inhibits their growth and/or multiplication. It might be thought that the latter is not as good as the former, but the inhibition provides a better opportunity for the host's immune system to respond to more-deadly infections. We also describe antibiotics as having either a broad or narrow spectrum. The former can affect many different types of pathogens, probably because the specific function they inhibit is common to all of them. However, the latter targets either only one type of pathogen or a narrow group of them. Although we cannot discuss the reasons behind these differences, the various mechanisms of inhibition elucidated have shed new light on basic metabolic processes of all bacteria. Another important concept is the use and need for multiple antibiotics. In particularly severe infections, or in immunocompromised patients, the chance that the pathogen can escape complete destruction is decreased considerably if several antibiotics are used. In addition, the possibility for the selection of resistant mutants is also decreased. The phenomenon of "synergism" comes into play here, which occurs when the effects of one antibiotic enhance the effectiveness of another, so that both together are more effective than either by themselves.

Interestingly enough, many of these drugs can also be toxic to host cells as well. Thus, it is important to choose the "right" antibiotic, which will be more effective against the pathogen than the host cells it was designed to protect. This requirement becomes even more of a problem when it is essential to use multiple antibiotics (as discussed above), which could have many side effects. Yet, obviously, there are many such antibiotics in use today, but they have to be applied judiciously. Nevertheless, the ideal antibiotic would be one that targets a metabolic function in bacteria that does not exist in animal cells. Do they, in fact, exist? Yes, and the best of them is one that has been around for the longest; namely, penicillin (produced by a fungus, *Penicillium notatum*) and its many synthetic and natural derivatives that have been developed over the years. These antibiotics target enzymes involved in synthesizing an important bacterial structure, the cell wall, which is vital in maintaining the cell's shape and exposure to the external environment and which animal cells (us) do not have. Of course, even these miracle drugs have bad side effects, such as developing fatal allergies to them (for which each patient should be tested before prescription), and there are many resistant pathogens now that are unaffected by penicillin.

Although we discussed the genetic mechanisms for antibiotic resistance, what exactly is involved on a metabolic level? There are three general mechanisms, which include the following: (1) a bacterial enzyme adds a "side chain" or a chemical structure to the antibiotic to physically prevent it from acting on its target, (2) the bacteria express an enzyme that actually destroys the antibiotic—again using penicillin as the example, many bacteria produce penicillinase (or beta lactamase), which when exposed to penicillin chemically degrades it, and (3) the antibiotic is prevented from being incorporated by the bacterial cell. In effect, the pathogen literally pumps it out before the antibiotic can penetrate the inner part of the cell (cytoplasm). Of course, there are variations on all these themes for resistance, and some pathogens display some or all of them.

Many important problems remain, which we broached only slightly, but clearly there are several outstanding ones. Some of them include (1) a search for novel antibiotics that target parts of pathogenic metabolism not targeted by others as well as toxin formation, which may not inhibit growth but will inactivate this most important virulence factor, (2) developing chemically stable antibiotics (so many are unstable in the body) that prevent pathogens from attacking them, (3) combining the use of antibiotics with completely different types of inhibitors for synergistic effects, and (4) searching for antibiotics that inhibit pathogenic fungi and protozoa, which hardly exist at all. Further reference to antibiotics will be provided in specific sections concerning specific pathogens.

5

Case Histories

A. Introduction: Why Are the Following Examples Chosen?

Now that we have discussed a wide variety of topics related to microbial pathogenicity and vibrant fields of knowledge encompassed in disciplines such as molecular biology and genetics that have helped us understand microbial behavior, we are ready to embark on a new journey. This journey will, I hope, enable us to explore in depth a number of infectious diseases caused either by a single microorganism or virus, or those caused by specific groups of microorganisms, so that as many different aspects of their causes and mechanisms of action as possible will be elucidated. In turn, it is hoped that this knowledge will spark an interest in your mind to explore further the byways and pathways of this vitally important era of "Microbes" and their profound effects on humanity. The problem, as always, is which infectious diseases to choose, because there are so many of them that have affected us in the modern era. Nevertheless, there are some, which seem to have affected us more than others or are more frightening to us, that stand out. These include HIV-AIDS, tuberculosis, influenza (human, avian, and swine), streptococcal and staphylococcal infections, cholera, and ulcers (caused by a most unusual pathogen called *Helicobacter*). However, there is another topic that involves diverse groups of microorganisms, viruses, or their products and that have been designated as possible bioterror weapons, which we also must discuss in depth to separate myths from realities.

B. HIV-AIDS: The Plague That Threatens Modern Society

In 1979, a new or emerging disease called acquired immunodeficiency syndrome (AIDS) appeared first mostly in homosexual males in the United States. **67**

Within a decade, the disease reached epidemic proportions, affecting the lives of millions of people all over the world, dominating health news and politics and forcing a redirection of medical research itself to determine its cause. The AIDS epidemic is a plague that has threatened modern society. However, it was quickly determined that it is not a disease of homosexual males only but can also affect women (40% of the total are now women) and children. It can be passed from an infected mother to her unborn fetus and can also be transmitted by contaminated needles and syringes in the drug culture, as well as by unsafe sexual practices. Tragically, contaminated blood has also been a culprit, infecting unsuspecting individuals by transfusions as well as those needing blood products, such as hemophiliacs. Most of the worldwide cases today are found in sub-Saharan Africa and Southeast Asia (although India has become a rapidly expanding focus) because of the lack either of treatment or education, or the failure to overcome social customs. From 1995, when semiaccurate statistics were assembled by the World Health Organization, through 2007, the number of cases has risen from fifteen million to thirty-three million. It has been calculated that a new case occurs every twelve seconds. And, according to a 2008 United Nations study, at least three people die of the disease every minute. It is the fourth leading cause of death in the world today behind heart attacks, strokes, and pneumonia. To be sure, other diseases such as malaria and tuberculosis affect more people than AIDS does, but the lack of a cure or a vaccine makes AIDS very alarming, even though there are promising drugs to treat the syndrome. This lack is very discouraging because researchers probably know more about the disease in terms of its cause—the human immunodeficiency virus (HIV)—than any other virus in history. It is probable that from the name of the disease and its cause, you can discern that the immune system of the host is compromised or destroyed. In fact, AIDS is one of a number of immune deficiency disorders.

1) ORIGINS

Before we proceed, however, it is of interest and importance to determine where in fact AIDS came from. First of all, it is a zoonoses that was transmitted from animals (probably chimpanzees that are infected with a similar virus) to man in East Africa about 60–100 years ago, and for many years it remained fairly isolated, with a limited spread among inhabitants of rural villages because of a stable lifestyle. However, this zoonoses is unusual because further transmission from the new host (mankind) to members of the same species can occur by the societal factors mentioned above. Second, when such societal factors disrupted this isolated lifestyle, AIDS spread to urban centers due to a disruption of family life and other factors, including poverty, increasing prostitution, and drug use. Third, there are many accounts of how AIDS spread from there to the United States and other Western nations, but they are speculative and do not provide additional insights into the syndrome. However, because AIDS is a sexually transmitted disease and is spread by contaminated blood, public education campaigns aimed at reducing transmission have helped to do just that, even in Third World countries. Thus, the use of condoms, micro-biocides (antiseptics that are used topically), sterile needles, and syringes has had some success, but in a limited way. New drugs (not antibiotics) have had more success, but in order to describe how they affect the primary cause of AIDS, the HIV virus, we must discuss this virus in some detail, including its molecular biology, because treatments rely on a succinct knowledge of such biology. It should be pointed out, however, that according to a World Health Organization report, anti-HIV drugs reach only approximately three-quarters of a million of the nearly seven million poor people in the world who most urgently need treatment. Thus, it is not only a matter of developing new drugs but of their low-cost distribution as well.

2) CHARACTERISTICS

The human immunodeficiency virus (Figure 5.1) is classified in a special group called "retroviruses." It is truly unusual in many respects. First of all, it is a spherical virus whose genetic material (genome) is made up of RNA—not DNA—and not just one RNA macromolecule, but two of them (both single

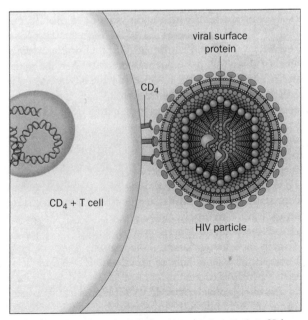

FIGURE 5.1 Infection by HIV. Sketch of how viral surface proteins attach to CD4 receptors in the first step of infection. A CD4 $^+$ T cell is a lymphocyte, a type of white blood cell involved in managing the production of antibodies. (See Plate 16)

stranded). These two RNAs are encased in a "nucleocapsid," a protective shell in the shape of a cone made up of one structural protein that surrounds the RNA genomes. Imagine something as "primitive" as a virus having two genomes, in comparison even to a much-larger and more complex bacterial cell that has only one (even though they are much smaller).

This "diploid"-like fact renders the virus much-more versatile than would be expected, as we will see later. Secondly, attached to the RNA genomes are special enzymes that are used by the virus to synthesize new RNA molecules, to process new viral proteins that are synthesized after infection, and to help it integrate itself by recombination into specific regions of the host's chromosomes. However, you might question how the RNA genome can integrate itself into a host chromosome that contains DNA as its genetic material, since if that were to occur, chromosomal DNA would become chemically unstable. Well, it does not! Instead, that is the function of the first enzyme mentioned above, attached to the RNA genome, called "reverse transcriptase." One of the most remarkable and unusual enzymes ever discovered, it seemed to violate all principles of the flow of genetic information "from DNA to RNA (mRNA) to protein," as we have discussed previously in an introductory section (see chapter II, sections D and E). One of its three parts (subunits, as they are termed) uses the RNA macromolecule as a template-substrate to synthesize a complementary DNA copy of itself (RNA "makes" DNA). Next, the second and third subunits chemically remove the RNA part of the DNA-RNA double-stranded hybrid complex and direct the still-intact complementary DNA strand to re-synthesize an exact DNA copy of the original RNA genome. It is this double-stranded DNA helix that becomes integrated by recombination into precise sites in the host chromosome, which then, by the normal processes of protein synthesis, employs host enzymes to transcribe the DNA and synthesize new viral proteins and RNA for its own propagation.

The nucleocapsid mentioned above is itself surrounded by a matrix of proteins that compose the outer shell of the spherical virus, which in turn is protected by an envelope of lipid (fat). This lipid-protein coat becomes very important in shedding the complete virus after it has been "manufactured" by assembly of its various parts. As if that complex structure weren't enough to marvel at, the coat also contains numerous "spikes" that are vital for attaching to specific receptor sites on the surface of the host cells it infects, primarily (although there are other kinds) a type of white blood cell called a lymphocyte (Figure 5.1). But as we will see, it is a special type of lymphocyte (termed a T-helper cell) that augurs badly for the immune system. The amazing fact is that the host receptor site itself (which is composed of two components known as CD4 and CXCR4, although other designations exist as well, such as CCR5) is vital for interacting with other host components that activate it, which are similar in structure and composition to the spikes on the virus. How such a remarkable feat of evolution occurred is unknown. Nevertheless, the entry of

HIV into the lymphocyte is actually assisted by the two components mentioned above. During this process, the lipid coat of the virus fuses with the lipid surface of the cell (or the cell membrane) because it is actually derived from that of the host. This fusion brings in the cone-shaped nucleocapsid core of the virus into the body (cytoplasm) of the lymphocyte, which is then degraded by enzymes to free the two RNA genomes (see Figure 1.7a in chapter I). It is at this juncture that reverse transcriptase performs its remarkable feat of synthesizing a double-stranded DNA copy (called cDNA), as described above. It then rapidly enters the nucleus of the T-helper cell and with the help of the HIV integrase enzyme (also mentioned above) becomes incorporated into the host chromosome by recombination. The cDNA thus becomes a permanent part of the T-helper cell's DNA, replicating with it at each cell division and remaining there for a decade or more, exactly like a lysogenic relationship between a bacterial phage DNA and a bacterial chromosome. At any time after integration, HIV genes can be activated by signals from the immune system along with the host's DNA to start gene expression by transcription and translation, and that is when the virus begins its own development. For this process, it uses all the host's transcription factors as well as some of its own, including one called *tat* that helps to speed up the entire process of transcription. Other viral transcription factors important to later processes of viral "maturation" and replication include *nef*, *rev*, *Vif*, and *Vpr* (Table 5.1).

An interesting question and perhaps a dilemma is which RNAs expressed by the viral genome are used to make new viral RNA chromosomes and which are used to code for new viral proteins and transcription factors? Obviously, to express a complete new viral genome the entire viral chromosome integrated into the host chromosome has to be synthesized. Thus, there has to be some kind of control exercised over gene expression. However, it turns out that this control is expressed after the entire viral genome is transcribed into RNA, by having some RNAs remain as they are (to serve as new chromosomes), while others are cut by a remarkable process termed "splicing" (discussed previously in chapter II, section E) to serve as messengers for viral proteins. Splicing in

TABLE 5.1

HIV accessory gene products

Gene Product	Function
Tat (transactivating protein)	Regulates transcription of genes that code HIV proteins
Rev (regulator of viral expression)	Binds to unspliced RNA transcripts and targets them for passage out of the host cell nucleus
Nef (negative factor)	Regulates HIV replication
Vif (viral infectivity factor)	Aids viral infectivity; role in virion assembly
Vpr (viral protein R)	Aids virus replication
Vpu (viral protein U)	Aids virus budding and release from host cell

the HIV virus is activated by the protein product of the *rev* gene mentioned above. Yet, these viral proteins are not the final end product—they require further processing by the protease enzyme that was bound to the RNA chromosome from the original infecting virus to yield the finished protein. All that "remains" is to package or assemble the RNA genomes into a cone-shaped nucleocapsid structure that forms, while the newly made viral surface proteins and the spikes are assembled at the surface of the cell. Somehow, the spikes attach to the nucleocapsid cone, and thousands of the viruses bud off from the infected cell after enveloping themselves like a shroud with part of the host's membrane, helped by another of the virus's gene products, called *Vpu*.

3) VERSATILITY

We will return below to a discussion of the existence of a seemingly large number of genes for what is presumably a very small virus. However, the "sophistication" of this "simple" life form does not stop there. To make it more difficult for the immune system to cope with the infection, HIV practices what we have described previously for some pathogenic bacteria; namely, "phase variation," the phenomenon whereby surface proteins are altered by a difference in gene expression. If you remember, by randomly switching on and off certain genes coding for surface proteins, antibodies that were generated by the infected host against the earlier proteins of the pathogen became ineffective against the later ones and had to be generated all over again (which takes time). In the case of HIV, the enzyme that synthesizes the cDNA copy of the RNA genome, reverse transcriptase, is the culprit. In an extraordinary insight, the enzyme is naturally defective in that when it copies the RNA strand into its DNA copy, it makes mistakes in pairing the purine and pyrimidine bases (for every adenine in RNA, a thymine should be its complement in DNA, whereas for a cytosine, it should be guanine). Actually, up to ten incorrect bases out of about eight thousand may end up in each cDNA synthesized. You might expect that this is bad for the virus, since the changes should be lethal. Although a majority of the genetic changes are lethal, few of the modified isolates emerge that have an advantage in replicative ability, because they produce different surface proteins that protect them. These new surface proteins force the immune system not only to generate a whole new set of antibodies but also to render some drugs ineffective as well. In yet another significant enhancement of viral evolutionary diversity that affects the immune system negatively, the fact that there are two complete RNA genomes can lead to recombination (mixing, remember?) between genomes of cells that are infected with two different viruses. That is, it is possible for the complete RNA transcripts from each of the integrated viral chromosomes to be encapsulated into a single nucleocapsid. When the complete virus (called heterozygous) infects a new cell, the reverse transcriptase enzyme can literally jump back and forth between the two different RNA templates, so that the newly synthesized cDNA sequence is a mixture (recombination) of genes not present in the original parents. This recombination increases the flexibility of the copying errors made by the reverse transcriptase enzyme mentioned above. The immune system, thus, has to face a multitude of new surface targets for which it must generate antibodies. Such recombination has resulted in the spread of naturally occurring recombinant virus strains to different parts of the world, where multiple variants exist. One such recombinant viral strain, for example, has spread to millions of persons in Southeast Asia.

4) STRUCTURE OF GENOME

An important insight we pointed out above was that an inordinately large number of genes are present in what is usually known as a "simple" organism (Figure 5.2, Table 5.1). In fact, without these genes, HIV would certainly not be the dreaded scourge it has become.

In order to understand how it is possible for the virus to express such complexity, a brief discussion of the genetic "structure" of HIV and its classification is necessary. The retrovirus group in which HIV is classified has RNA genomes and three gene loci (sites), which express three main functions. These include (1) the *gag* locus, which controls the expression of proteins involved in synthesizing the nucleocapsid core proteins, (2) the *pol* locus, which controls expression of enzymes involved in synthesizing the RNA genome (reverse transcriptase), guiding the cDNA into the host's chromosome (integrase) and processing viral proteins that are produced (protease), and (3) the *env* locus, which controls the expression of enzymes involved in synthesizing the spikes and their subsequent fusion with the cell membrane. However, we mentioned six additional genes that are not found in the gene loci just described, such as *tat*, *rev*, and *nef*, among others. Where are they located? In an incredible example of viral "ingenuity" (a number of viruses do this, by the way), the same segment of integrated viral DNA can be utilized to code for different proteins than they normally would (as described for the three loci above), by beginning translation at a different codon (remember this term; see chapter II, section E) within that segment. The different start sites are produced by differently splicing the long, complete mRNAs after transcription. We call these genes "overlapping," and, as implied, they enable a relatively short sequence of bases in a viral chromosome to code for "more than they are entitled."

5) TREATMENT

Besides the intrinsic value of elucidating as many aspects of HIV's virulence as possible through molecular biology and genetics, such information, as pointed out previously, is vital in designing drugs to treat or, one hopes, cure the disease

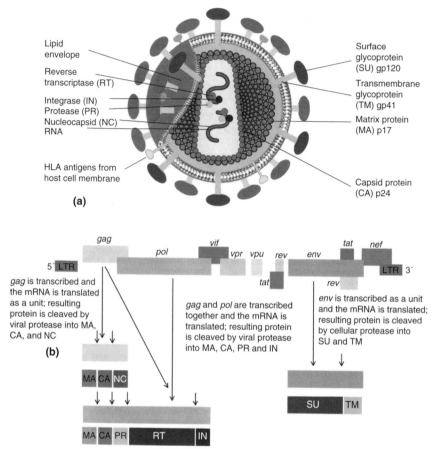

FIGURE 5.2 Human immunodeficiency virus, type 1 (HIV-1). (a) Diagrammatic representation of the virus, showing important protein antigens. (b) Map of the HIV-1 genome, showing its nine genes and flanking long-terminal repeats (LTRs). The LTRs contain regulatory sequences recognized by the host cell. (c) HIV-1 gene products. The accessory gene products are translated into proteins of final size, while *gag* and *pol* products must be cleaved by viral protease, and *env* products by host cell protease. The small arrows indicate the sites of cleavage. (See Plate 17)

that ultimately leads to AIDS. In general, there are thirteen distinct steps in the life cycle of HIV (which were described above) for which a possible drug target could be designed to disrupt. Of course, like for antibiotics, it is vital to develop drugs that affect the virus but not the host. One of the earliest and most important anti-HIV therapies was developed in the 1990s, called HAART (highly active antiretroviral therapy). This consists of multiple drugs (a "cocktail," as it is known) that target two main activities of the viral life cycle at different stages. The first group inhibits the synthetic activity of the reverse transcriptase enzyme that synthesizes a cDNA copy of the RNA genome. Perhaps you have heard of AZT, an anticancer drug that was found to inhibit the formation of the reverse transcriptase enzyme, but there are now a number of others as well that inhibit the activity of any or all of the three subunits that make up the enzyme, or that bind to them. The other group of inhibitors acts to inhibit the activity of HIV's proteases, which are essential in processing the viral proteins made late during development. The principle behind such cocktails is that although the virus might develop resistance to one or even two of the inhibitors, it is unlikely that it will be capable of becoming resistant to all of them at the same time. In fact, the impact of these cocktails on victims of AIDS has been dramatic and has led to the first real decline in deaths from AIDS in the United States, from 50,000 in 1995 to less than 20,000 in 2000. Tragically, the cost and distribution of these multiple drugs make them less available in regions that still suffer greatly from AIDS, such as sub-Saharan Africa and Southeast Asia. We do not have the time and space to discuss the many brilliant ideas that have been put forth for new types of therapies, but they are absolutely amazing in their insights. You may get a sense of what these therapies are by reading the science sections of most newspapers and magazines periodically.

One major type of treatment that should be the one of choice, as it is for most viruses, is vaccination. You might find it unusual that currently there are no approved vaccines for preventing HIV infection. Yet, attempts to develop vaccines against HIV were initiated soon after the disease became recognized. Their failure thus far, despite enormous investments in time and money, underlines which host cells are targets for infection—namely, those of the immune system itself—although other cell types from the brain, kidney, liver, and heart can also be infected, but at reduced rates. We cannot discuss the various types of immunity that a vaccine should induce (active or passive). Nevertheless, in order to understand the mechanism of HIV infection, some aspects of immunity are necessary to describe in more detail.

6) COURSE OF INFECTION

When HIV infects its host through the various methods we described earlier (unsafe sex, contaminated syringes, needles, or blood), it can enter a number of different cell types from the immune system, depending on the particular HIV strain and host cell. However, the most important one is a type of white blood cell we described earlier, called T-helper cells or CD4 lymphocytes. There are several types involved in inflammatory reactions and in controlling the expression of many of the properties of the immune system. In a sense they act as the "traffic cop" at a busy multiple-entry junction, directing the various cell types of the immune system to be processed or developed further, which occurs after any infection to produce circulating antibodies or special kinds of lymphocytes that kill infected host cells by direct contact. Thus, you can suspect that by interfering with the activity of this T-helper lymphocyte or by destroying it, the immune system itself can be brought down. However, it can take up to ten years before this destruction is expressed completely. Nevertheless, the initial infection acts like most others. The immune system is activated (including T-helper CD4 lymphocytes) by the virus (called an antigen), and amazingly enough, most but not all of the entire infecting virus is destroyed (Step 1). Flulike symptoms may occur while the infection spreads throughout the body. As the virus decreases, the activated immune system and levels of the CD4 lymphocytes decrease too, "satisfied" that the job has been accomplished. This occurs over a period of about two to three months. However, virus levels slowly start to increase while the levels of the CD4 lymphocytes increase only slightly, but not nearly to the levels observed in the primary infection, and then slowly they start to fall despite the supposed stimulation by the HIV antigen (Step 2). Probably this is due to infection of new CD4 cells by the virus, although it does not seem that there is a great level of infection and CD4 cell destruction. Interestingly enough, it is during this phase that drug therapies have the best effect in treating, but never curing, the infection. This period has been called asymptomatic and can last for up to eight years, the only symptom being swelling of the lymph nodes (those sites in the body where the white blood cells are concentrated to interact with their antigens, and a junction between lymph fluid and blood). Slowly but surely, the number of CD4 lymphocytes, which is normally about one thousand per microliter (a very small volume of liquid) of blood serum, is decreased to less than fifty per microliter, while the number of viruses increases even further. It is at this juncture that full-blown AIDS is manifested (Step 3). The immune system can no longer cope with this infection or, indeed, many others that opportunistically infect the host. We will describe them and other maladies below. Symptoms include vast lymph node enlargement, weight loss, fever, diarrhea, and, finally, death. In fact, the end game occurs in the lymph nodes, the intense site of antigen interaction with the lymphocytes, which start to degrade and release their "detritus" (viruses, lymphocytes, other white blood cells, etc.) into the blood circulation. Some types of infected white blood cells called macrophages can circulate into the brain and cause great destruction there, resulting ultimately in dementia. Incredibly enough, what kills most victims is not HIV but infection by opportunistic pathogens. Indeed, some of them are so unusual that their frequency in the early 1980s led doctors to suspect a newly emerging disease. We cannot list them all, but they include tuberculosis (both human and bird), legionella pneumonia, measles, typhoid, yeast brain meningitis, herpes simplex, toxoplasmosis (a protozoan disease), and a type of pneumonia that is the leading cause of AIDS deaths, caused by a very small bacterium called *Pneumocystis carinii*. Malaria (caused by a protozoan) also figures prominently in the AIDS pandemic in an unusual way, in that it stimulates the production of the CD4 lymphocyte cells that are targeted by HIV. This stimulation causes greater replication of the virus, resulting in much-higher death rates of those co-infected with both pathogens. Thus, malaria may be a deadly cofactor for HIV in places where they both exist, such as sub-Saharan Africa. Another insidious manifestation of AIDS is the development of cancer. It has long been suspected that cancer arises because of failures in the immune system, and AIDS certainly belongs in this group. One of the earliest cancers that was recognized in AIDS victims was called Kaposi sarcoma, a cancer that affects the skin and internal organs. Apparently the cancer is induced by an AIDS-associated virus related to the herpes virus, whose different types can cause a variety of infections—from the "cold sore" to genital infections and possibly cancer. I make this point to illustrate how, even out of the tragedy of AIDS, research can reveal new phenomena that would not have been discovered, in this case the existence of another virus that may cause cancer.

7) CONCLUSIONS

Despite our extensive discussion of HIV and AIDS, there is much that we have not discussed, such as natural resistance to AIDS by certain groups of people, new factors involved in virulence of HIV, novel methods of treatment, new methods of education about AIDS that involve special groups of individuals who are at high risk, and special problems for health workers, among many others. Nevertheless, it is certain that the discussion we did have should provide a greater understanding of what is probably the most dreaded plague of the twentieth and twenty-first centuries.

C. Tuberculosis: The White Plague, Ancient, But Still Lethal

1) INTRODUCTION

Many people in our modern society do not believe that tuberculosis is of importance in their lives. Of course, they have heard of this dreaded disease, but not many know of anyone who has it. In truth, this belief is not unreasonable, because tuberculosis has declined in the industrialized world over the past hundred or so years, due to great improvements in our living conditions. Nevertheless, this "opinion" is naive and dangerous. In fact, despite such lifestyle improvements, a significant part of the population probably has a positive response to diagnostic tests (discussed later) for the microorganism that causes it (*Mycobacterium tuberculosis*). That is, at one time in their lives, they were exposed and infected by the pathogen, which can easily be passed between individuals by coughing or sneezing, just like a cold, but fortunately their immune system responded positively to the infection and destroyed it. It is an amazing fact that approximately 95% of all human beings with normally functioning immune systems are resistant to developing the disease, but it is that remaining 5%, which is still a significant number, that is the problem. In addition, this latter population has grown because of pandemics such as AIDS and multiple antibiotic-resistant tuberculosis organisms. Known since antiquity (mummies from ancient Egypt have shown symptoms of tuberculosis), the disease has had a profound effect on human history and evolution. Famous operas such as *La Boheme* (where the heroine dies of tuberculosis), and the description of the disease as the "white plague" for many centuries, attest to its fearsome reputation. Here are some sobering statistics. (1) Over the past two centuries, over one billion people have developed tuberculosis. (2) Tuberculosis is the leading cause of death in the world from a single infectious disease. (3) Eight million new cases of tuberculosis are detected every year, of which 20% are now resistant to multiple drugs and antibiotics. (4) In the United States, there are approximately ten million Americans living with the disease. Because it is spread so easily, the prevalence of tuberculosis depends on the living conditions of a community. Thus, societal factors such as poverty, inadequate nutrition, unsanitary living conditions, and overcrowding are pivotal in this regard. Another prime factor in susceptibility to tuberculosis involves debilitation of the immune system. Such debilitation can be a result of other disease such as AIDS, smoking, working in mines, and genetic defects. Finally, the prevalence and mortality of the disease jump precipitously in the so-called Third World or developing countries. For example, babies are often infected and harbor the microorganism for many years until the disease becomes manifested in young adulthood. Without treatment, which is often the case, most of these young adults die.

2) DESCRIPTION

If viewed by microscopy (Figure 5.3), the tuberculosis organism (TB for short) resembles a long, slender rod that when subjected to various diagnostic tests can be separated from "true" bacteria because, among other properties, its surface has an unusual structure that is very rich in lipids (up to 60% of the entire content of the organism itself, much higher than other bacteria), which actually promotes virulence. Known as the cord factor (because TB colonies form long, cordlike structures), it is a waxy substance consisting of lipids that are complexed with sugars (known as glycolipids).

Mutants of TB that do not contain the cord factor are not pathogenic, but its mechanism of action is still unclear, although it may be involved with survival after engulfment (phagocytosis) by special white blood cells called macrophages. In a sense, it acts like an "endotoxin" (that part of the surface of many bacterial pathogens, described in chapter I section D, that is responsible for virulence, but the chemical and structural compositions of each is different). One unusual characteristic of TB is that it grows very slowly, much less so than normal bacteria (twenty hours doubling time, compared to twenty minutes). Thus, it would seem that TB should be more vulnerable to various

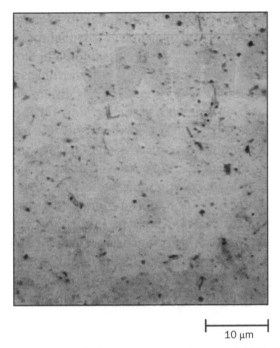

10 µm

FIGURE 5.3 *Mycobacterium tuberculosis* as seen in sputum from an individual with tuberculosis. The sputum has been "digested," meaning it has been treated with strong alkali to kill the other bacteria that are invariably present. (See Plate 18)

drugs and antibiotics. Yet, it is precisely this unusually slow growth rate that causes many practical problems, because therapy has to be sustained for a long time and, also, standard methods of identification can require many weeks.

3) PATHOGENICITY

There are two main stages of infection, termed primary and secondary. In the primary infection, almost everyone who is exposed to TB, most commonly by inhaling the bacteria (as little as ten can be effective), will harbor the organism for a while, but, as stated above, most of those with normally functioning immune systems will overcome the infection and will destroy the pathogen. Only the activation of a specific kind of inflammatory factor that reacts with surface or other protein components of TB will attest to the fact that some individuals who required a certain period of time to overcome the pathogen were actually infected. However, in a minority of the population (mostly children or immunocompromised adults), this primary infection will develop further. Although TB can infect any organ in the body, approximately 85% of all the cases remain in the lungs. After about three to four weeks, the immune system mounts a furious reaction, whereby the TB organisms are localized

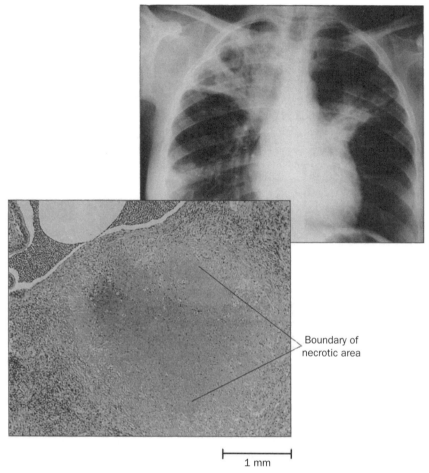

Boundary of necrotic area

1 mm

FIGURE 5.4 Stained lung tissue, showing a tubercle, a kind of granuloma caused by the body's reaction to *Mycobacterium tuberculosis*. The innumerable dark dots around the outer portion of the picture are nuclei of lung tissue and inflammatory cells. Centrally and extending to the right of the photograph, most of the nuclei have disappeared because the cells are dead, and the tissue has begun to liquefy. The photograph depicts a chest X-ray film of an individual with tuberculosis.

to remarkable structures in the lungs, called tubercles (Figure 5.4). These are massive complexes that contain a number of different kinds of immune cells and other components such as the protein collagen (which makes up bone cells) that form a wall (or "prison") around the TB organisms so that they cannot escape. Although the TB bacilli are still alive, they remain dormant as long as they remain within the tubercles.

Such tubercles can remain for a long period of time in the individual, with little outward symptoms as long as their immune systems are function- ing even at a slightly reduced rate. However, if left untreated, victims begin to experience more-severe symptoms such as coughing up blood, fever, difficulty in breathing, a type of allergy that destroys tissues (see below), and loss of weight. It is this gradual weakening of the body that accounts for older characterizations of the disease as "consumption." Approximately 50–70% of these people will ultimately succumb if not treated.

The sequence of events that establishes the infection in the lungs is at once fascinating and terrifying, because those very cells involved in destroying the infection, the macrophages, are compromised by the TB organism itself. The bacilli travel down the respiratory tract in droplets, and when they get to the lungs they are phagocytized by the macrophages in those areas of the lung, which exchange oxygen with carbon dioxide (called alveoli). However, instead of being destroyed within the phagocytes as most pathogens are, the TB organisms actually thrive because of several factors. They include the cord factor, which inhibits the destructive powers of the macrophage, and other incredible metabolic reactions induced by the pathogen, which prevent other destructive cell-toxic processes from operating. In effect, the TB organism actually stimulates the macrophage to engulf it by secreting factors that activate recognition factors from the host's immune system itself that identify a foreign "body" (antigen). As a result, the pathogen is protected after phagocytosis from other outside immune factors that could destroy it. Thus, in an analogous manner to viruses, the TB organisms metabolize host nutrients to replicate freely within the macrophages, gradually killing them, after which they can be engulfed by other macrophages that start the process all over again. This cycle does not mean, however, that the host's immune system is completely impaired. It continues to fight the ongoing infection vigorously. Eventually, an inflammatory process is triggered which results in the attraction of many additional macrophages and other types of cells to the lung to initiate the formation of the tubercles (as described above). This completes the "primary" stage of TB infection. In the secondary phase, there are two possible outcomes, one of which we described above as activation of TB after many years. Part of this activation involves the development of a type of allergy called delayed hypersensitivity in those individuals who form tubercles. Because of the lifelong persistence of the organisms, many different types of immune lymphocyte cells are also activated, among which are those that secrete inflammatory factors called cytokines, designed to stimulate immunity to TB by attracting large numbers of macrophages. Of course, these lymphocytes are "unaware" that is precisely what the TB bacillus wants—namely, to be phagocytized—although these cytokines can also destroy bacilli that have not yet been engulfed. Unfortunately, such inflammatory factors also damage many kinds of tissues internally and externally over a long period of time, which contributes to the progression of the disease. The second "secondary" response is termed "disseminated" tuberculosis, which is a direct extension of being infected initially. In this more devastating form of the disease, which occurs mostly in children or debilitated (immunocompromised) persons, the TB organism is spread throughout the body with the formation of very small tubercles in many organs, but without any delayed hypersensitivity because of its swift progression, which leads to death very quickly. It should be pointed out that disseminated TB can also occur in those individuals who have developed active TB after many years.

4) TESTING AND VIRULENCE FACTORS

There are a number of classic tests for detecting whether TB may or may not be present or, rather, whether there is evidence that the individual has been infected previously. However, that is precisely the problem, in that it takes time (up to six weeks) to definitively demonstrate whether the TB organism can be cultured from the infected individual. During this period, the infected individual can spread the disease to others. The classic tests include chest X-rays of the lungs to directly visualize tubercles or other damage (Figure 5.4) and the so-called tuberculin or Mantoux test, which can also provide presumptive evidence. Of course, chest X-rays, when numerous, are by themselves harmful to an individual, so it is not the most ideal test. The Mantoux or tuberculin test, which is less damaging, involves injection of a small amount of a protein derivative of TB itself (called PPD) under the skin. After forty-eight to seventy-two hours, a delayed hypersensitive reaction will occur in the skin, as detected by the formation of a small bleb if a positive reaction is indicated. Examination of the bleb shows a heavy infiltration of macrophages and lymphocytes. For both of these tests, any positive result will signify only that the test subject was previously exposed to TB, but not that he or she necessarily has the disease. Recognizing the need for faster diagnostic methods, sophisticated techniques in molecular biology have been developed that show great promise and allow the detection of the pathogen within two weeks instead of six. Another problem is the difficulty of studying the effect of infection and onset of the disease in human beings because of ethical considerations. Yet, there are few animal models that are available, since the human form of TB can be duplicated accurately only in primates. Thus, understanding virulence factors and their expression and developing vaccines and useful drugs and antibiotics are not simple tasks. What works in the typical animal models such as mice, rabbits, and guinea pigs does not translate very well to human beings, although there have been advances, since such models have been used for more than a century. Yet, mice do not develop tubercles, guinea pigs are much more susceptible to TB than are humans, and rabbits are resistant to human TB but susceptible to a form of TB that infects cattle (*Mycobacterium bovis*). This latter infection has proven useful to study, since the organisms can also cause TB in immunocompromised patients or in individuals who consume raw milk that has not been pasteurized. Nevertheless, not many virulence genes have been identified, and new animal models have been sought. One unusual and unconventional success, according to M. Trucksis, a professor of microbiology at the University of Maryland, has been that of goldfish, where TB is caused by *Mycobacterium marinus*, a species that not only mimics many of the symptoms of human TB, such as the formation of tubercles and its ability to thrive in macrophages (at a much-faster rate), but whose genome is very similar to that of human TB. Many new mutants of goldfish TB have been isolated by Professor Trucksis in an attempt to enlarge the sparse number of virulence genes that have been identified, and, one hopes, to identify new targets that might be useful for developing a vaccine in humans.

Another approach has been to compare the genomes of human TB strains freshly isolated from infected hosts and those that have been maintained in the laboratory for a long time. Unfortunately, many studies of virulence for many pathogens have been carried out by using well-established laboratory strains. This has proven to be unwise because by not being in contact with their natural hosts, most pathogens have accumulated mutations and other changes that render them avirulent, or unable to cause the disease. Thus, in a comprehensive study of freshly isolated and laboratory strains of TB by a large group of researchers at several places in the United States, headed by Professor R. D. Fleischmann from the Institute of Genomic Research, in Rockville, Maryland, significant differences in genes involved in synthesizing cell surface components were found in the former that were not present in the latter. That is, the genes were present in the latter but they did not have the same genetic sequence of bases. Such differences in genes that perform the same function are called "polymorphisms" and are good candidates for virulence and immune determinants.

Thus, much remains to be understood with respect to the many virulence factors that TB uses to cause this most dreaded infectious disease. Researchers are still in the beginning phase. Nevertheless, treatments for TB have been among its most successful stories yet, as discussed below.

5) TREATMENT

Sometimes it is difficult to understand why tuberculosis is such a worldwide problem, because it is so treatable even in immunocompromised patients. At present, treatment usually involves administration of multiple antibiotics and other drugs for a sufficient period of time to kill the bacilli in the lungs and almost everywhere else in the body and to prevent the rise of resistant TB mutants. Unfortunately, a number of problems have surfaced, some of which we alluded to above. First, successful treatment requires from six to twenty-four weeks, often with individuals who are the most difficult to control, such as the poor, the indigent, and drug addicts, as well as AIDS patients. When the treatment is halted prematurely, resistant mutants start to proliferate in the host, and further treatment becomes impossible or much-more difficult. Second, common and cheap antibiotics such as penicillin have little effect on TB because they target the synthesis of structures (the cell wall) that are different in TB. Also, such antibiotics are cleared from the body before they can have a chance to react. Third, as pointed out above, TB is engulfed by macrophages rather quickly, which protects them from a number of drugs and antibiotics. Initially, the first "cocktail" of drugs developed consisted of streptomycin and rifampin (antibiotics that lyse [destroy completely] slow-growing TB bacilli), and isoniazid (a drug that is highly specific for all mycobacteria because it inhibits the synthesis of the cord factor). There are a number of other combinations that have been used when multiple drug-resistant (MDR) TB organisms surfaced because of negligence in maintaining treatment. This problem has become more severe even in some industrialized countries such as New Zealand, Denmark, Germany, and the United States. Between 10 and 20% of all TB cases are MDR, and epidemics are extremely costly to control, such as one in New York City in the 1990s involving AIDS victims, which cost over two billion dollars before it subsided. As a result, a number of programs and technologies have been proposed or developed, designed to ensure that patients take their proscribed "TB cocktails" or medications until the infection has been cured. The first is called DOTS (directly observed treatment short-course), where health-care workers observe patients continually to ensure they take their cocktails consistently. The second is an attempt to develop an implant impregnated with suitable drugs and antibiotics that would be placed underneath the skin and slowly deliver the agents into the circulation over a period of months.

It is important to point out that with all such cocktails there are problems with side effects, cost, and allergies that can severely affect a patient and must be considered when prescribing therapy. Finally, one of the most pressing problems is to discover new antibiotics or drugs that combat TB. It is difficult to understand that with all its deadly effects, the last really new TB drug was introduced in 1963. Since then, a few others have been developed but have not been tested against TB, except for one that is described below. We discussed in a previous chapter why many pharmaceutical firms are not actively seeking new drugs, which has to do with cost and with restrictions on their use to only one disease, such as TB. Therefore it is worth singling out Bayer (the aspirin maker) for its very generous offer to use their newest antibiotic, Moxifloxacin, as part of a contract with the Global Alliance for TB Drug Development, a public-private partnership to treat TB. Clinical trials started in 2005 involving thousands of patients in eight countries, including Brazil and Zambia, an exciting advance in controlling the disease.

You might be wondering whether a vaccine, which is probably the best course of prevention, exists. The answer is yes and no. In countries where TB is common (Africa, Asia) and where it isn't (Europe), many patients are immunized with a vaccine called "BCG," but not so in the United States. It is named after two Belgian scientists (Calmette and Guerin) who developed the vaccine by growing an attenuated (weakened) strain of a closely related TB organism that infects cattle (*Mycobacterium bovis*). It has been used to immunize thousands of susceptible individuals such as children and others in places where TB is rampant (such as in Africa). Unfortunately, there have been conflicting studies that show good protection against human TB or none at all. The vaccine has never been approved in the United States because (1) it interferes with the tuberculin test for TB (giving false positives) and (2) it can also cause TB in immunocompromised patients.

After almost eighty years of decline in the United States, a startling upturn in TB cases began to appear, especially in New York City during the middle 1980s, when such cases began to increase by about 5% a year until 1992, when a peak was reached with almost 30,000 new cases reported. Two factors played a role. One was the increase in the appearance of multiple drug-resistant strains, as discussed above, but the second was an alarming and more rapid progression of TB in AIDS patients. Instead of the slow course of TB progression over a period of years, TB infections progressed in a matter of weeks and months in such patients, resulting in the deaths of approximately 80% of the cases despite drug treatment (even if the TB organisms were susceptible). Fully one-third of all TB cases reported resided in AIDS patients. It was soon recognized that AIDS patients who had previously been infected with TB and had localized the organisms to tubercles were unable to do so effectively as AIDS progressed over the years and weakened the immune system. As a result, disseminated or reactivated TB ensued, with the bacilli spilling out into other parts of the lung and ultimately thriving in many organs all over the body. In other words, they did not need the "protection" of the macrophages because the entire immune system itself was wasting away. Another complication in AIDS cases or in any immunocompromised individual is that other strains of TB such as those that infect cattle (mentioned above) and even birds (*Mycobacterium avium*) are able to cause TB. Clearly, TB prevention and treatment remain at the top of any list in terms of cost, but more importantly, in terms of the misery it continues to cause to humanity.

D. Streptococci and Staphylococci: More Intimacy Than We Desire

1) INTRODUCTION

How many times have you heard of the characterization of a common microbial disease as a "staph" infection, or a "strep" sore throat? Many times, I will bet. Not only that, but there is hardly anyone who has not seen the actual manifestations of these infections in themselves or others, such as a pimple or an abscess in the former case, or a hacking cough, fever (sometimes), and an inflamed throat in the latter case. Actually, although you might not be aware of other infections caused by "staph" (known as staphylococci) or "strep" (known as streptococci), they are very common and sometimes very deadly. For example, impetigo (a contagious skin disease of the face or arms), osteomyelitis (an infection of part of the bone), scalded skin syndrome (another skin disease in which patches of skin slough off), toxic shock syndrome (known as STSS; internal infection resulting in severe shock), endocarditis (a heart infection originating from blood poisoning), and a type of food poisoning are all caused by different strains of staphylococci. Similarly, pneumonia; scarlet fever (which we discussed previously); rheumatic heart fever; tonsillitis; toxic shock syndrome, leading to a massive degeneration of the skin and, ultimately, internal organs (known as TSS, which we also discussed previously); and of all things, dental cavities, are examples of streptococcal infections. Yet, by no means have we exhausted the incredible list of assaults on human beings and other animals by these two genera. Why are they so prevalent and why consider both genera together? In order to understand their extraordinary pathogenicity, we will discuss their adaptability and their ability to produce numerous toxins.

2) GENERAL DESCRIPTIONS

Both groups consist of sphere-like bacteria that do not have organs of loco-motion (called flagella) but that can still move by being attracted or repelled by certain chemical stimuli. It is surprising that these organisms can cause so much potential damage, even though they are intimately associated with human beings. It might be expected that there is some kind of adjustment or adaptation to allow each to coexist without "harm" to the other, and indeed this is the case most of the time. However, some events occur that can predispose the host quickly to become susceptible. These include societal and other factors such as injury, poor hygiene and nutrition, other chronic infections, diabetes, and immune deficiencies, and specific factors such as the season (e.g., winter) or locales (e.g., hospitals). All humans become colonized almost as soon as they are born, which continues throughout life. A normal healthy adult carries the organisms on the skin, nasopharynx, and intestine. More specifically, depending on the season, between 5 and 20% of normal individuals carry potentially pathogenic streptococci ("group A" strep, see below) in their throats, which is why they are primed to cause pharyngitis (strep sore throat) and bronchitis (infection of the air passages leading to the lungs) mostly in the winter or spring. These usually are cleared up by the immune system unless some of the societal and other factors mentioned above are operative, which can then result in more deadly diseases such as scarlet and rheumatic heart fevers. Occasionally, such "group A" strep can cause the dreaded toxic shock syndrome mentioned above, by invading deeper tissues and organs. Nevertheless, up to 40% of normal individuals contain streptococci that inhabit the upper respiratory system, such as in the nose, but they are not as virulent except for one species that causes pneumonia. Staphylococci, on the other hand, are mostly associated with diseases of the skin because they are much more resilient than streptococci to extreme changes on this surface, such as salt (from sweat), acidity, dryness or desiccation, radiation (from the sun), and heat. This tolerance also allows them to exist on a variety of nonhuman surfaces as well. However, staphylococci can also be found in the upper respiratory tract, the intestine, and the urinary and genital regions as well. Let us now discuss each genus separately and in more detail to illustrate their amazing breadth and pathogenicity.

3) STAPHYLOCOCCI

It is relatively easy to distinguish staphylococci from streptococci, by two criteria. The first is the way in which both group themselves as they divide. Under the light microscope, staphylococci grow in grape-like clusters because they divide from "north to south" during one division, and from "east to west" in the next one (or vice versa). This ultimately results in irregular cell clumps, which do not separate from each other. In contrast, streptococci, in one of the wondrous sights of microbiology, grow in long, convoluting chains (Figure 5.5) that also do not separate, especially if nutrients are in short supply.

The other criterion is easily demonstrated by simply adding some hydrogen peroxide (bleach) to a liquid culture of either organism. If staphylococci are present, the bleach will bubble violently as it is chemically degraded into water and oxygen because of the presence of the enzyme catalase. This degradation will not occur in a culture of streptococci, because they lack the enzyme. Of course, there are other more sophisticated diagnostic tests that can be performed to distinguish not only the two main groups but different species within each group. Perhaps no other pathogen can produce as many virulence factors as do staphylococci, but no single factor can account for its overall virulence. Rather, combinations of many factors are operative. Yet, most researchers regard one particular virulence factor, the production of the enzyme "coagulase," as being most indicative of staphylococcal virulence, and when clinicians detect this enzyme in a diagnostic test, physicians are very concerned for the patient. In addition, it is produced only by one species of staphylococci out of the five such species that are important clinically; namely, *Staphylococcus aureus*. That is why it is known as the primary pathogen of humans and animals, the one commonly detected in abscesses. The enzyme acts by clotting the soluble host protein fibrin that is activated during the formation of clots, and it accumulates around the bacterial cells, making it difficult for white blood cells to phagocytize them. Yet, it also walls off the abscess to isolate it from the rest of the body, almost like a "tubercle" does in tuberculosis. If the immune system is functioning normally, the infection will eventually be overcome. The other four species are opportunistic pathogens and

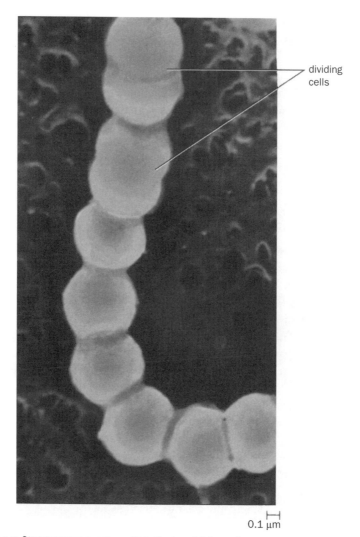

dividing cells

0.1 μm

FIGURE 5.5 *Streptococcus pyogenes*. Note the two dividing cells.

mostly cause problems in immunocompromised individuals, even though, as stated above, none of them produce coagulase. It is amazing that one of these opportunistic species, *Staphylococcus epidermis*, composes almost 90% of the bacteria that exist on the skin, whereas *Staphylococcus aureus* makes up most of the rest of the population. However, they both exist in the upper respiratory tract of normal individuals as well. In an important revelation concerning the presence of *Staphylococcal aureus* in nasal passages of different individuals, it seems that some natural populations are more virulent than others, regardless of the individual, sort of like a hierarchy of virulence. By modern techniques of genomics (sequencing the entire genetic makeup of each isolate), a pattern was found in which certain genes were disproportionately common in the "hypervirulent" isolates, but not in the less pathogenic ones. How is this possible, since they all are *Staphylococcus aureus* strains? Such subtleties are due to the random selection of certain traits that enable the organisms to become more "ecologically" fit for survival and virulence. Indeed, there was a strong correlation between patients with serious staphylococcal invasive diseases and the presence of these hypervirulent "clones." How they arose originally is unknown, but it does illustrate another of the many facets of pathogenicity to which humanity must adapt.

4) TOXINS

The many toxins produced by *Staphylococcus aureus* can be separated on the basis of whether they act as enzymes, which are destructive to tissues, or whether they act as true toxins that interact with specific cells or components of cells (Table 5.2).

The former group includes coagulase (already discussed above); hyaluronidase (also known as spreading factor because it dissolves the gluelike substance hyaluronic acid, which binds various host tissues together); staphylokinase, which actually dissolves blood clots (Can you think of a beneficial use for this enzyme? See below for a similar enzyme in streptococci); nucleases, which degrade both host DNA and RNA; and lipases, which degrade lipids and help staphylococci colonize oily skin surfaces. The latter group, which all are classified as exotoxins, includes two types of hemolysins (which destroy red blood cells), leukocidins (which destroy white blood cells or phagocytes), two exfoliative toxins (which destroy skin or epithelial cells), several enterotoxins (which destroy intestinal cells and activate nerve cells that cause the cramping, vomiting, and diarrhea characteristic of food poisoning), and, finally, the incredible toxic shock syndrome toxin or STSS (which induces

TABLE 5.2

Properties of *Staphylococcus aureus* implicated by its virulence

Virulence Factor	Action Site	Action
Clumping factor	Bacterial surface	Attaches bacterium to fibrin, fibrinogen, plastic devices
Fibronectin-binding protein	Bacterial surface	Attaches bacterium to acellular tissue substance, endothelium, epithelium, clots, indwelling plastic devices.
Protein A	Bacterial surface, extracellular	Competes with Fc receptors of phagocytes; coats bacterium with host's immunoglobulin
α-toxin	Extracellular	Makes holes in host cell membranes
Leukocidin	Extracellular	Kills neutrophils or causes them to release their enzymes
Enterotoxins	Extracellular	Superantigens. If systemic, causes toxic shock; causes food poisoning if ingested
Toxic shock syndrome toxin-1	Extracellular	A superantigen. If system, causes toxic shock.

high fever, shock, and rapid destruction of at least three organ systems). It is useful to elaborate further on some aspects of their formidable activities. For example, the two main types of hemolysins, which destroy red blood cells, can be detected (and differentiated) quite readily on solid nutrient medium to which red blood cells have been infused. As the cells grow into visible colonies or clones, they secrete each type of toxin, which produces two zones of hemolysis. The first zone, closest to the colony, which completely destroys (lyses) the red blood cells, producing a clear area, is mediated by the so-called alpha toxin. A second zone, which diffuses farther away from the colony and results in a fuzzy, incomplete destruction of the red blood cells, is mediated by the so-called beta toxin. Why the organism requires two such toxins or has evolved to produce them is unknown, but as with all redundant or semiredundant reactions that microorganisms exhibit, it may be to compensate for the loss of one of them by mutation or other genetic mechanisms. This "requirement" may also be the case for some other toxins, such as exfoliating toxins A and B that are involved in scalded skin syndrome, and the four enterotoxins that are involved in food poisoning. There is another type of multiple activity where two different toxic substances act "synergistically" (remember this term from our discussion of antibiotics, where two or more antibiotics act more efficiently than either by themselves?). Thus, coagulase, the definitive virulence enzyme produced by *Staphylococcus aureus*, covers the bacteria with host fibrin (the clotting substance) to prevent phagocytosis. If, nevertheless, the bacteria are still phagocytized, they secrete the toxin leukocidin inside the white blood cell, which destroys them from within by disrupting the cytoplasmic membrane. In fact, as you probably know, dead phagocytes make up most of the pus that is observed after a staph skin infection. Finally, perhaps the most incredible and deadly toxins of all are those that cause toxic shock syndrome (STSS in staphylococci and TSS in streptococci). Strictly speaking, such toxins are not directly toxic to a specific cell or cell component. Rather, they compose a class of proteins (in bacteria and viruses) that induce a massive stimulation of the immune system, by activating many different kinds of T-lymphocytes that are absolutely essential as the first responders to foreign substances (antigens). (Remember the several types of T-lymphocytes that are activated in HIV-AIDS infection? See part B of this chapter.) In fact, up to 70% of the total number of T-cell types involved in these responses to antigens are activated. Only in this case, the immune system is fooled because there aren't numerous different infectious antigens assaulting the host, but only one or a very few that have been labeled by Professor P. Schlievert of the University of Minnesota and others in the late 1980s as "superantigens" or SAgs (see Figure 1.5 in chapter I). By stimulating such large numbers of T cells, massive levels of inflammatory cytokines are also secreted by the activated T cells (also discussed previously in the chapter on tuberculosis), resulting in the TSS and STSS syndromes of high fever, delayed hypersensitivity, and interference with the liver's ability to clear normal poisons. Although we cannot discuss in detail the complicated mechanism by which this large activation occurs, SAgs act by binding to a receptor on the surface of many different kinds of T cells to activate them. As such, they are nonspecific in contrast to more-conventional antigens, which activate one in about ten thousand T cells instead of one in five. In addition, whereas conventional antigens are "cleaved" on the surface of the T-lymphocyte during further processing, the SAgs are not. Thus, they can keep on functioning. There are a number of additional deadly ramifications of SAg action, such as causing autoimmune diseases in which the body starts to react to its own proteins and other components. Rheumatoid and other forms of arthritis and rheumatic heart fever may be examples of autoimmune diseases caused by SAgs. It is difficult to imagine how these small, one-celled creatures can induce so much harm to humans and animals, but they do. Now, let us discuss the diseases themselves in more detail.

5) STAPH DISEASES

Most staphylococcal diseases begin as a local skin infection that progresses in severity. If not treated or cured, the infection can either develop further because the bacteria are able to access the circulatory system, where they can spread throughout the body to cause blood poisoning (bacteremia), or it can become localized again in specific organs and tissues. The skin infections are called "cutaneous" lesions and usually start as a minor abrasion, although they can also begin naturally through skin glands or hair follicles. The first significant manifestation is called an abscess (or a furuncle), where the bacteria penetrate "subcutaneous" layers underneath the skin surface. Perhaps the best metaphor is a "war" to describe what transpires. An intense "battle" begins, characterized by the attraction of large numbers of "warriors" from the host's side (macrophages, other white blood cells called neutrophils, and T-lymphocytes) to the site of infection. At the same time, "enemy troops" (*Staphylococcus aureus*) increase their rate and extent of multiplication, secreting toxins that destroy phagocytes and red blood cells and producing coagulase that deposits fibrin around their cellular surfaces to inhibit further phagocytosis. Meanwhile, T-lymphocytes have started the process of generating antibodies, by inducing another lymphocyte (B) to differentiate into plasma cells and by producing inflammatory cytokines, which is manifested by an increased redness of the area around the abscess, the probable rupturing of the abscess, and the escape of pus. As more and more of the phagocytes and bacteria are destroyed, macrophage reinforcements arrive, attempting to engulf everything in sight. These include disintegrating fragments of their own kind, red blood cell fragments, and disintegrating bacteria. This is the crucial stage. If the immune system is going to prevail, the furuncle gradually decreases in size, redness (inflammation) also decreases in size, and the entire area hardens from deposited fibrin. If, on the other hand, the pathogen prevails, multiple furuncles begin to form subcutaneously, which penetrate farther beneath the skin. The area of inflammation increases dramatically, and swelling and rupture into surrounding tissues often occurs. Such a deep lesion that spills over into surrounding tissues is called a "carbuncle." However, it is important to point out that these events are predicated on the lack of treatment and subpar immune system. Antibiotic treatment (provided the patient does not harbor antibiotic-resistant staphylococci) is safe and very effective in combating the infection, even in immunocompromised individuals. Another common staph skin infection is impetigo, a very contagious disease whose symptoms include small, flat, red patches on the face and arms or legs. A terrible affliction of young children whose immune systems have not yet developed fully, these patches often erupt, producing pus and eventually forming a scar or crust that itches mercilessly. The infection can spread internally to the lymph nodes, resulting in inflammation and further pain. This disease is called erysipelas and can be fatal if not treated. Lastly, scalded skin syndrome is a disease primarily of infants, in which the outer skin actually starts to separate or peel off from lower layers, a condition that spreads all over the body, producing large blisters. It can last up to ten days but is not fatal unless secondary infections by other pathogens occur. Nevertheless, it is a frightening phenomenon for mothers to witness on their babies.

Regardless of the initial source of staph infection, it is highly likely that further invasiveness will occur systemically (without treatment), producing either a bacteremia (blood poisoning) or localized diseases such as osteomyelitis, a chronic infection of the bone. This disease is very common among athletes and in young children who have had sports-related or other injuries. Perhaps the most famous of them was the star centerfielder of the New York Yankees, Mickey Mantle. The symptoms are marked by fever, chills, pain, and muscle spasms. In its most common form, the staphylococci spread in the circulatory system, enter the artery that supplies blood to the bone, and lodge in the small vessels of what are called "bony packets." Growth of the bone cells causes inflammation and swelling. Sadly, in many instances of athletic endeavor, the weakened bones break. Other systemic infections can occur in the lungs (staph pneumonia), a very debilitating disease with fever, chest pains, and bloody sputum. Only a small percentage of cases are due to this infection, but they are 50% fatal if not treated. The invasion of the circulatory system can also lead to heart infections (endocarditis) and meningitis (infection of the lining of the brain). In the latter case, 15% of all meningitis cases are due to *Staphylococcus aureus* instead of the more well-known meningococcus organism. Although we mentioned staph food-poisoning organisms, it is worth pointing out why it is the most common of all food-poisoning organisms. This is due to the fact that the toxins can be expressed in as little as two hours after food has been contaminated. Almost any food that is left out for a short period of time (such as at picnics, weddings, and bar mitzvahs), even when treated with salt, can be affected. There is no odor to indicate that the food has been contaminated, nor is there any change to alter its taste. Fortunately, the poisoning is rarely fatal and lasts between twenty-four to forty-eight hours. Nevertheless, you will know that you have been infected "big time"!

6) TREATMENT

Although humans have a strong resistance to staph infection due to their immune defenses, despite the many virulence factors described above, resistance to antibiotics, particularly the penicillins, has become a big problem. Staph is notorious for acquiring resistance quickly, and they continue to defy attempts at control, primarily because of the lack of antibiotics. It is a "given" that evolution will inevitably produce resistance to the common antibiotics used today, as well as the few new ones that have been discovered. Therefore, it has become essential (1) to develop rapid diagnostic assays to ensure that the antibiotics that are used are effective, and (2) to use multiple antibiotics to make it less likely that resistant mutants will arise. Nevertheless, as long as humanity survives, there will always be staph infections and those people who carry staph asymptomatically. Perhaps the best and simplest way to control such infections is to pay careful attention to hygienic practices (e.g., washing hands, disposal of contaminated material properly, and wearing surgical masks).

7) STREPTOCOCCI

Although streptococci are not as robust as staphylococci, they are as devastating for the numerous diseases they cause, primarily of the respiratory system. As with staph, there are a number of important species clinically, and a large number of them were initially characterized in 1935 by a famous immunologist, Rebecca Lancefield, who at the Rockefeller Institute devised a classification based on immunological reactions. Four groups were delineated, with the most virulent being group A, which contained over eighty "serotypes" (or Lancefield surface antigens) of *Streptococcus pyogenes*, the primary cause of pharyngitis (sore throat), scarlet and rheumatic heart fevers, and kidney disease. They produce (among many other toxins) hemolysins, which induce the clear (beta) type of red blood cell lysis. As a result, when a streptococcal disease is identified as "beta hemolytic group A streptococcus," physicians know that the dangerous *Streptococcus pyogenes* is present and that it is time for significant antibiotic treatment if the infection does not clear up by itself. Of the three remaining groups, one of them (group B) contains species that can cause an invasive meningitis in infants (*Streptococcus agalactiae*), while group C species are opportunistic pathogens that can cause sore throats but do not lead to further damage. The last group (D) is the only one containing nonpathogenic streptococci. There are many other streptococcal species that lie outside these four main groups, including the dreaded organism that causes the majority of all cases of pneumonia (*Streptococcus pneumoniae*), another species that causes a severe case of endocarditis (heart infection) (*Streptococcus viridans*), and still another that has an important role in causing dental cavities (*Streptococcus mutans*).

What seems to be unique in the group A streptococci, besides their exotoxins, is the large number of structures on its surface that contribute to virulence (Figure 5.6). These include attaching "organelles" (mentioned previously in an earlier chapter) called fimbrae, which are found in many other pathogens but which in streptococci are made up of unique proteins called "M proteins" that may have multiple functions, including inhibiting initial stages of sensitization by components of the immune system, leading to their lysis.

There are over eighty different kinds of M proteins, making it difficult for the immune system to react against individuals infected with more than one type of *Streptococcus pyogenes*. Other proteins include two that also help "strep" attach to host cells such as fimbrae (called protein F) and inhibit phagocytosis (called protein G). As if that weren't enough, there is a capsule composed of hyaluronic acid, the sticky substance found in all of us that helps maintain the integrity of our connective tissue. It is amazing that the same acid composes the capsule of *Streptococcus pyogenes*, helping it to resist phagocytosis but, perhaps more important, disguising the bacteria so that the host's immune system does not recognize it as a foreign antigen (or has trouble doing so) because it is a normal component of the body. There are still other structural components that act as antigens (called the group-specific carbohydrate antigen) to induce specific antibodies, which place *Streptococcus pyogenes* in the group A category. What their main function is in *Streptococcus pyogenes*, other

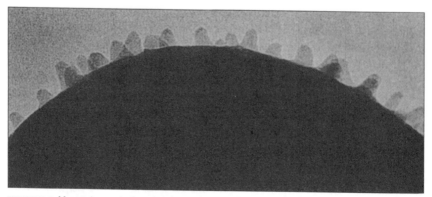

FIGURE 5.6 M proteins and other proteins of the cell surface of a *Streptococcal pyogenes* cell that help it combat the immune system.

than that characterization, is unknown. Nevertheless, to clinicians, they are a valuable diagnostic marker. Recently, through the use of the modern technology of genomics, as many as fifteen new proteins have been identified on the group A streptococcal surface, which has not only demonstrated its incredible complexity but has indicated a whole new approach to understanding how the pathogen invades many tissues. The reason is that they are "multifunctional" in their ability to interact with host proteins. That is, they bind to different types of antibody proteins in the serum or other environments (such as saliva) and also act as enzymes to break down unrelated host components such as a type of cholesterol. Although there is no explanation yet for such multiple activities, it may be that they are important as sensory signals for the bacteria to indicate where they have been "deposited," such as in an environment enriched in one type of antibody but not another.

8) TOXINS

Like staphylococci, the many toxins produced by streptococci can be differentiated on the basis of whether they act as enzymes or specific poisons. The enzymes include those that degrade host DNA and RNA, a protein-cleaving enzyme called C5 (a peptidase that helps the M proteins mentioned above inhibit processes by the immune system, designed to sensitize the bacteria for eventual lysis), and an enzyme that dissolves fibrin (called streptokinase), the clotting substance that may impede the bacteria from spreading into other tissues because it forms around capillaries and other blood vessels. In addition, the formation of fibrin signals the production of local inflammatory factors that could destroy the streptococci. Without fibrin, inflammatory factors are not produced as readily. So, imagine the miracle, if you will, of using this enzyme in the treatment of heart attacks! An individual who suffers a heart attack does so in many instances because of the formation of a fibrin clot in the arteries leading to the heart, especially the coronary artery. Heart specialists realized that if the clot could be dissolved within a few hours of its formation, the victim would have a good chance of survival. One of the ways this has been accomplished is by injection of streptokinase directly into the blocked artery. And it works! Go figure. A similar enzyme is produced by staphylococci, but for a number of reasons the streptococcal enzyme is preferred. As for the major severe protein toxins of streptococcus, they include streptolysins O and S, which destroy not only red blood cells (that characterizes their "beta" hemolysis), but also leukocytes (white blood cells) and liver and heart muscle cells, by rupturing their cell membranes. Another deadly toxin (actually a family of them) is pyrogenic (fever inducing) and causes a multitude of diseases, including pharyngitis (strep sore throat), which can lead to scarlet fever and ultimately heart and kidney traumas (rheumatic heart fever and glomerulonephritis). However, others in this family (which are not necessarily initiated

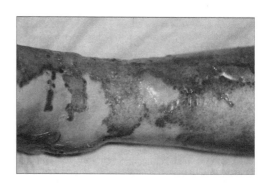

FIGURE 5.7 Individual with *Streptococcus pyogenes* "flesh-eating disease" (necrotizing fasciitis).

by a sore throat) are responsible for the dreaded toxic shock syndrome (TSS) discussed earlier in this section, which destroys vast areas of the skin rapidly (called "flesh-eating" necrosis) (Figure 5.7).

In addition, as also pointed out above, all these exotoxins are superantigens that induce massive levels of inflammatory factors because they activate the T-lymphocyte part of the immune system. Although we have discussed the complications of the strep sore throat above and previously in the chapter on emerging diseases, it is useful to describe them in more detail here, "fortified" with our knowledge of the organism itself as a bacterium. The strep sore throat, which can be extremely painful and differentiated from a viral infection by the high fever it causes, can lead to serious complications in two stages. The first is scarlet fever, caused by the pyrogenic (high-fever) toxin, which also produces a red rash all over the body. The toxin is released in the throat and enters the bloodstream, circulating throughout the body. The disease lasts about ten days, sometimes causing another infection of the tonsils in the form of an abscess. Occasionally, long after scarlet fever has ended, the second stage can manifest itself, either causing rheumatic heart fever (which damages the valves of the heart so that they leak) or damaging cells of the kidney so that they cannot adequately filter blood, resulting in swelling, increased blood pressure, and low urine output. In either case, long-term debilitating effects can occur, resulting in a heart "murmur" or kidney failure. The actual mechanisms of the toxic effects are not completely understood but may involve a number of possibilities; namely, continued or new infection by the streptococci, continued or new secretion of the superantigen exotoxins, continued or new activation of inflammatory factors produced by T-lymphocytes, or a combination of these factors. Nevertheless, the actual number of first- and second-stage cases has declined over a period of many years, due to effective antibiotic treatment and the possibility that the genes producing the pyrogenic toxin itself may have weakened during evolution or may have been transferred to a different strain of group A streptococci, resulting in the new TSS syndrome. This latter possibility was discussed extensively in chapter IV, on emerging diseases.

9) OTHER STREPTOCOCCI

Three other pathogenic streptococcal species not included in the group A–D classification also exist and continue to cause humanity great problems. Two of them are involved in diseases of the gums or in the formation of dental caries (cavities). The first, *Streptococcus viridans*, is a normal inhabitant of the gums, which can be "activated" by dental procedures that lead to injury of the gums or by the formation of an abscess in the mouth. As an opportunistic invader, the organism can enter the circulation and lodge in the heart, producing a "subacute endocarditis," or in the lining of the brain, producing meningitis. The second is *Streptococcus mutans*, an important inhabitant of the tooth surface that ferments sugars to produce a slime-like acid end product called plaque that coats the enamel surface of the tooth and eventually erodes it. It is important, however, to point out that there are numerous nonstreptococcal species that colonize the mouth, as you can imagine, that are also involved in tooth decay and gum disease, as well as many others that help to control the potential pathogenic types. Finally, one of the most deadly of all streptococcal species that lie outside the group A–D classification is *Streptococcus pneumoniae*, the primary cause of lobar (lung) pneumonia (Figure 5.8). It is one of the few streptococcal species that do not form long, convoluted chains but instead exist as "diplococci" (in twos) surrounded by a polysaccharide capsule.

We have also discussed its importance medically and genetically in previous chapters, but as a disease, it knows few equals in its ability to devastate

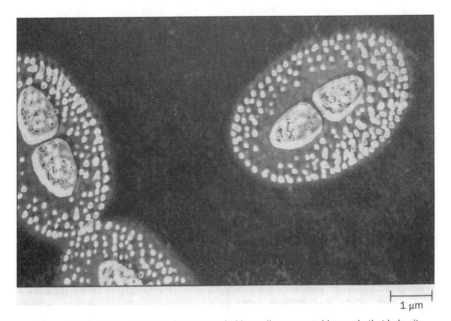

1 μm

FIGURE 5.8 *Streptococcus pneumoniae* surrounded by a slippery mucoid capsule that helps it avoid phagocytosis.

victims, accounting for approximately 70% of all those that must be hospitalized. The pathogen is a normal inhabitant of the nasopharynx and travels down the trachea to the lungs when a host becomes "susceptible," due to a variety of societal and other factors mentioned previously. Those most vulnerable include individuals with poor or underdeveloped immune systems (such as the old and very young, and AIDS patients). The bacteria lodge in the air sacs (alveoli) of the lungs, causing a severe inflammation resulting in bloody sputum, severe chest pains, and severe difficulty in breathing. There are more than ninety-two different types of pneumococci, all of which are based on differences in the structure and composition of the polysaccharide capsule surrounding the cells. The capsule is a primary virulence factor because its presence inhibits phagocytosis, while noncapsulated pneumococci are avirulent. However, only four or five of the types are responsible for most human pneumonia. Pneumococci also produce a number of toxins that lyse red blood cells (such as pneumolysin), but their complete range is still unknown. What is important is the deadly growth cycle that occurs to propagate the bacteria in the lungs. As they grow, toxins are secreted, damaging or destroying cells and releasing important growth factors into the microenvironment of the lungs, which the pneumococci exploit for their own metabolism. Among the most important of these growth factors are precursors for DNA replication, which the cocci incorporate into their cells to stimulate further growth. Further multiplication results in greater secretion of toxins, which damages and destroys additional cells, releasing DNA precursors to start the cycle all over again. Of course, the body tries to limit the growth of the pneumococci by generating antibodies and other substances to attack them. Before the advent of antibiotic therapy, which is still relatively successful, there was a deadly race between the rapidity in which the immune system could be harnessed to fight the disease, and the cycle of virulence. The patient had to lie still and not exert himself or herself for a significant period of time, until the "crisis" was past, which was usually signified by profuse sweating and a reduction of fever. Pneumonia is also an example of a disease that occurs seasonally, mostly in the winter and fall, although healthy individuals are very resistant to the disease.

E. Ulcers and Helicobacter: The Uncommon Pathogen

1) INTRODUCTION

Almost the entire adult population on Earth experiences some type of stomach inflammation (called gastritis). This discomfort can be occasional or chronic and can range from mild to severe indigestion (heartburn) to mid- and upper abdominal pain itself. Many foods and beverages and other substances can cause these debilitating effects, including alcohol, coffee, and aspirin. The prime host culprit is, of course, stomach acid, which is required to digest food so it can be absorbed ultimately into the bloodstream through the small intestine. In a significant number of cases, it was commonly believed that the production of too-much acid, as well as the action of inflammatory factors, could aggravate the stomach lining and the lining of the part of the small intestine closest to the stomach, called the duodenum, leading to gastric ulcers. Such ulcers are typified by depressions in these linings, resulting from too-much gastric acid secretion, which destroy the cells and membranes of which they are composed. In severe cases, perforations in the linings can occur, causing bleeding, and/or disgorging contents into the body, causing great and deadly harm. As bad as perforation of the stomach or intestinal lining, the development of one of the most common cancers worldwide (gastric adenocarcinoma) and a type of lymphoma (cancer of lymphocytes that produce antibodies) are also a possibility in about 20% of ulcer cases. For most of the twentieth century, treatment of gastritis and ulcers lay in various anti-acid medicines and anti-inflammatory drugs. Such anti-acids and new ones, which suppress the production of stomach acids, are still used for treating mild cases of indigestion. However, the gastritis world was turned upside down in 1983, when two microbiologists from Australia, B. J. Marshall and J. R. Warren, discovered a strong association between gastritis and the presence of a small, curved, rod-shaped bacterium called *Helicobacter pylori* (Figure 5.9a).

The discovery was striking because not many microbiologists believed that any bacteria could grow in the human stomach. Nevertheless, these two microbiologists not only were able to culture the organisms from stomach acid and gastritis and ulcer patients, but one of them, B. J. Marshall, in the grand tradition of early microbiologists in the early part of the twentieth century, swallowed a culture of the pathogen, giving himself a severe case of gastritis. Fortunately, gastritis is rarely fatal, and he treated himself successfully with antibiotics to demonstrate that the condition could be cured. This revolution was so significant in challenging the prevailing dogma—that gastritis was a physiological disease rather than an infectious disease—that they were awarded the Nobel Prize for medicine in 2005. In addition, their discovery has led to consideration of how other chronic "physiological" conditions such as arthritis and certain kinds of heart diseases may actually be triggered by pathogens.

2) THE ORGANISM

In considering how the organism survives and proliferates in stomach acid, the pathogen is not "so stupid." Of course, it cannot grow free in the extreme acidity of the stomach (Figure 5.9b). Instead, cleverly, it sequesters itself in the mucus layer secreted by special cells that line the stomach, and in the intestine (called epithelial cells), which is less acidic. Another "trick" it has evolved is the secretion of an important enzyme called urease, which converts urea to ammonia to help neutralize stomach acid in the microenvironment. Urea is

Overall structure of Helicobactor pylori

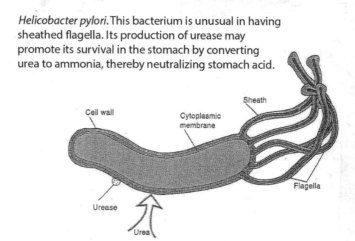

Helicobacter pylori. This bacterium is unusual in having sheathed flagella. Its production of urease may promote its survival in the stomach by converting urea to ammonia, thereby neutralizing stomach acid.

How gastric ulcer formation is caused by Helicobacter pylori

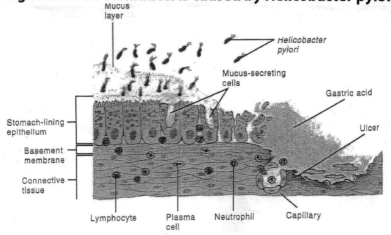

FIGURE 5.9 (a) Overall structure of *Helicobacter pylori*. (b) How gastric ulcer formation is caused by this organism.

a byproduct of protein catabolism of the cells that secrete the mucus. In fact, the production of excess ammonia not only is toxic to the epithelial cells but also results in less-complete digestion of food and the occurrence of halitosis (bad breath) in infected individuals. One difficult problem is how *Helicobacter* travels to the mucus layer during initial or subsequent infections. It must be exposed to the full force of the acid, as well as to strong enzymes such as pepsin and trypsin, which are present in the stomach and help digest food proteins, but which could also affect proteins of the pathogen itself. Possible but only partial answers include the presence of a number of powerful organs of locomotion (which we have mentioned previously for other pathogens) called flagella. These flagella are clustered at one end of the bacterial cell (called polar), so that when the bacteria move they seem to be "jet propelled" and penetrate the mucus like a corkscrew. In addition, they are protected, unlike many other flagella, by a thick protein sheath to resist digestion by stomach acid, as well as possible proteolytric digestion by the stomach enzymes. However, there are no clear answers to this conundrum. A more detailed discussion of infection and *Helicobacter*'s many remarkable virulence factors will be given below.

3) THE DISEASE

It is a fact that 75% of patients with gastric ulcers and 95% of patients with duodenal ulcers are infected with *Helicobacter*. This can be easily tested by a procedure known as endoscopy, where a probe is introduced into the stomach through the mouth, pinching off a small piece of the stomach lining, which is then assayed for the presence of urease. Further tests can be performed to culture the organism if the urease test is positive. The important questions are how do we become infected and does the presence of the organism always signify ulcers? It is amazing that *Helicobacter* is a normal inhabitant of almost one-half the world's population, and almost 100% in developing countries. In the United States, the organism is found in about 30% of adults but in over 65% of elderly individuals, more in lower socioeconomic groups. Since only approximately 15% of those infected develop ulcers, the implication is that most of us harboring the organism are asymptomatic; that is, we will never develop ulcers, and in some cases, their presence early in life may even be helpful, as described below. So why do ulcers erupt? It could be, for example, that a particularly virulent strain is the cause, one that produces an array of strong toxins, since there is a huge diversity of different *Helicobacter* strains that have been isolated that infect both humans and animals. Another possible factor may be at what age an individual becomes infected. Although it is true that *Helicobacter* has probably infected humans and their ancestors for hundreds of thousands of years, there is a correlation between the percentage of individuals infected and their societal niche. The more "difficult" the niche (such as in developing countries or lower socioeconomic groups), the greater number of individuals who are infected early. Nevertheless, this early exposure permits the immune system to develop partial immunity to their presence, which may help ameliorate the development of ulcers, in contrast to those in upper socioeconomic classes who may not be exposed to the organisms until later in life. As a result, such latter individuals would be less tolerant to an initial exposure and more prone to the disease. We discussed a similar societal problem in the chapter on emerging diseases (chapter IV), in the case of polio. The ease with which *Helicobacter* can spread probably accounts for its almost universal infection rate. Many carriers, such as houseflies, can contaminate food simply by landing on it after a life cycle in which the bacteria are present in the substrate that housefly eggs are laid on (e.g., human or animal feces).

4) PATHOGENICITY

To further explore the mechanisms by which *Helicobacter* causes ulcers, we begin by following its passage into the inhospitable stomach acid. Already mentioned above were the roles of the powerful flagella in guiding the bacteria into the mucus layer secreted by epithelial cells of the stomach lining, and in the production of ammonia from urea, both of which reduce the level of acid. Another mechanism to counter stomach acidity that may be important during the "journey" to the mucus layer is the presence of "transporter" genes, which express products that literally pump out any excess acid that tries to enter the vulnerable cytoplasmic portion of the organism. However, the bacteria need to maintain themselves once they arrive at the mucus layer against the natural processes of digestion, such as flushing (peristalsis) of the gastric contents. The flagella help by "swimming" against the tide of flushing, but the bacteria must also be able to stick or bind to some receptor sites on the epithelial cells as well. This is accomplished by the presence of adhesins (glue-like protein components, which were discussed in a section of the introductory chapter as essential virulence factors of many pathogens), which enable them to adhere to mucus and epithelial cells. The best-defined adhesin is a surface protein called BabA, which binds to a number of red blood cell surface proteins that comprise the common ABO blood antigen groups (existing in all humans), and others related to type O that are also found on the surfaces of intestinal epithelial cells. In fact, type O individuals are much more susceptible to peptic ulcers, suggesting that binding of the BabA adhesin of *Helicobacter* to the O-like receptor is involved in the severity of this disease. In yet another remarkable adaptation by *Helicobacter* elucidated by a group of Swedish and French scientists, resistance to constant attack by macrophages and other phagocytes that try to engulf them is thwarted by a transient switching of the genes that express the surface adhesin proteins such as BabA, which is the primary target of such phagocytes. Instead, other surface adhesins, which can also bind the antigens, are expressed (called SabA) that are not recognized well by the phagocytes. What triggers the switching in response to the proximity of the phagocytes is as-yet unknown. However, this type of "frustration" could lead to extraordinary chronicity of *Helicobacter* infection, as discussed further below.

5) TOXINS

Like so many other pathogens, *Helicobacter* produces a combination of enzymes and toxins that account for its virulence. For the former, we have already discussed urease, which not only is important for providing less acid environment by producing alkaline conditions, but such alkalinity is also toxic to the epithelial cells aiding in their destruction. However, the production of large amounts of urease may have another unintended function, namely to activate and attract cells (lymphocytes) that produce inflammatory factors like cytokines. Many others exist. However, it is precisely the repeated attempts by inflammatory cells and their cytokine products to destroy *Helicobacter* in the protected environment of secreted mucus (along with the genetic switching phenomenon described above) that may contribute to constant irritation and long-term damage of the stomach and intestinal lining. The lymphocytes and other white blood cells have difficulty in penetrating this layer, as shown by their relative absence, but their products are present in gastric epithelium cells. Two other enzymes, catalase and superoxide dismutase, are also probably important in helping *Helicobacter* resist phagocytosis. One of the most important correlations between severity of ulcers and *Helicobacter* is whether or not they produce two protein toxins. One is called VacA (first described in 1988 by Robert Leunk at the pharmaceutical company Proctor and Gamble), which destroys cells from within (a cytotoxin) and produces the lesions characteristic of gastric ulcers when injected into mice. The other is called CagA, which probably expedites translocation of VacA into the cells. There are fascinating correlations between the presence or absence of these two toxins, how much of each is expressed, whether mutations have resulted to impair their functions, and the severity of the disease, which suggests strongly that they are the prime "movers and shakers" of *Helicobacter*. First of all, approximately 50% of *Helicobacter* isolates fail to produce VacA activity, although a protein that is very similar to VacA is still detected, suggesting that one or more mutations have occurred to render the protein inactive. Second, approximately 40% of *Helicobacter* isolates fail to produce CagA. In this case, either the protein itself is not produced, or, like VacA, a protein similar to CagA is expressed but inactive. Most important is that its presence strongly correlates with expression of VacA cytotoxin activity. In many investigations, almost 100% of *Helicobacter* isolates expressing VacA activity also produced CagA. However, CagA activity could still be detected in about 25% of *Helicobacter* isolates that did not express VacA. In summary, therefore, the following conclusions were reached: (1) VacA cytotoxin production of *Helicobacter* isolates is consistently greater in peptic ulcer patients than in those with simple gastritis (heartburn, indigestion). (2) Almost 100% of patients with duodenal ulcers also express the CagA protein in *Helicobacter* isolates, as compared to 30% with gastritis only. (3) When both VacA and CagA genes are expressed by *Helicobacter* isolates, a much-greater inflammatory response occurs (which destroys gastric epithelium cells) than in those that express only one or the other gene products. Thus, (4) the greatest clinical impact occurs when both VacA and CagA are actively produced by *Helicobacter*. Nevertheless, other virulence characteristics still have to be taken into account, such as whether urease is produced as well, since *Helicobacter* mutants lacking this protein have been isolated and are not pathogenic.

Needless to say, long-term damaging effects by inflammatory factors in chronic sufferers may lead to the two cancers mentioned in this chapter's introduction (a gastric adenocarcinoma and a lymphocyte lymphoma). Such cancers claim hundreds of thousands of lives a year, especially in developing countries whose citizens are also heavily infected with *Helicobacter*. In a fascinating recent study, two scientists from the University of Massachusetts, J. M. Houghton and T. Wang, have suggested that *Helicobacter*-induced inflammation of the gastric epithelium cells also attracts bone marrow stem cells (which can differentiate into many types of cells). However, in this case, such stem cells try to repair the lining of the stomach but, due to the devastating long-term inflammation, are not normal and develop into cancer cells instead. This work is still controversial, but it has led to new investigations concerning inflammation and cancer. One interesting and important confirmation of the role of inflammation has come, of all places, from AIDS sufferers, where the opposite occurs; that is, the depletion of the immune system results in a lower incidence of damage and fewer cases of ulcers. New developments in genomics, in which the entire *Helicobacter* genotype has been decoded, have led to the detection of new genes that may be involved in virulence. In fact, these studies have revealed that approximately only half the total number of *Helicobacter* genes have been uncovered.

6) TREATMENT

Although *Helicobacter* is sensitive to many antibiotics and other drugs, and its successful eradication would surely help in decreasing the cancers described above, the organism is still difficult if not impossible to eliminate from the "gut." Such difficulties are due to the degradation of antibiotics by stomach acid and enzymes, flushing or diluting them after ingestion, difficulty of penetrating the mucus layer, and, of course, development of natural resistance of *Helicobacter* through evolution. Nevertheless, ulcers can be treated by these agents by using a multiple regimen, which includes antibiotics such as ampicillin (a derivative of penicillin) and bismuth compounds (which are available over the counter as "Pepto-Bismol"), as well as methods to prevent flushing and chemical degradation. Treatment lasts approximately three weeks, with a 90% cure rate.

In conclusion, the past fifteen years have seen substantial progress in research on this unusual pathogen, which causes so much misery in so many people. Although much more is required to elucidate further aspects of virulence, it is hoped that its susceptibility to treatment with well-known antibiotics and drugs will alleviate much of this misery within a decade or two.

F. Cholera: A Pretty Nasty Beast

1) INTRODUCTION

There is a famous "saying" that cynically cites two certain events that plague all humans; namely, "death and taxes." To those two certainties, however, I would add a third event: gastritis, or "stomach ache." There is little doubt that every human being (and animal) on this planet suffers from gastrointestinal upset at one time or another. There are almost as many causes as there are people, ranging in severity from "hardly noticeable" to "life threatening." Most causes are not so dangerous, but some are, such as being infected by a number of different pathogenic microbes. Three of them are very well known and include typhoid, cholera, and dysentery. Their abilities to cause disease are due to specific toxins that they secrete, which act on epithelial cells in the small or large intestine and ultimately cause a severe diarrhea that can cause dehydration and death. Moreover, secondary "insults" to the body, such as kidney failure and blood poisoning, can also occur. Most of the time these secondary effects arise as a result of people or animals drinking fecally contaminated water, although passage of the disease by direct contact can sometimes occur from contaminated food. Nevertheless, it cannot be spread from person to person like a cold or influenza can. Although any of the three diseases could have been chosen for further insights, I have decided on cholera because it is constantly in the news, and because there have been so many outbreaks over the past few decades (the latest in Haiti). According to the World Health Organization (WHO), there are an estimated three to five million cases and 100,000 deaths due to cholera reported each and every year, mostly in resource-limited nations.

Since the early nineteenth century there have been seven cholera pandemics. Hundreds of thousands of people died in these early outbreaks because of the lack of treatment, and even when such treatments were discovered (rehydration and antibiotics), it was still difficult to control them—mainly because so many people were infected so quickly. Nevertheless, the death rate has decreased (but is still significant) compared to the early pandemics, because of knowledge gained and aggressive treatment.

2) THE ORGANISM

Cholera is caused by an innocuous organism (*Vibrio cholerae*) that looks like a "comma" under the light microscope (Figure 5.10), as if the rest of its form (a corkscrew) were abruptly cut off.

The original habitat for the organism (most of which are avirulent; that is, nonpathogenic) lies in the coastal areas around the globe, in association with zooplankton (microscopic animal organisms that float in the oceans of the world) and algae in freshwater areas (Figure 5.11).

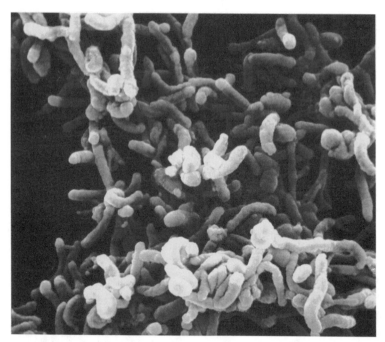

FIGURE 5.10 Electron microscope photo of *Vibrio cholerae*, showing its comma-like morphology.

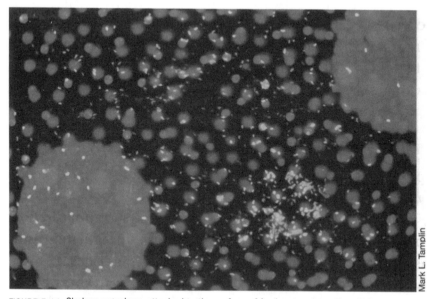

Mark L. Tamplin

FIGURE 5.11 Cholera organisms attached to the surface of freshwater algae. The cholera organisms are stained green. The red color is due to the fluorescence of chlorophyll A in the algae. (See Plate 19)

When the zooplankton or algae multiply because of warm weather conditions, they can reach huge numbers together with their vibrio "tenants." So the question remains: How did the pathogenic strains arise from the nonpathogenic strains and become so deadly? The answer revealed by scientists in the 1990s is an exquisite example of lysogenic conversion, which was discussed in chapter II, section G (Genetic Modifications). It is defined as an alteration in the properties of a microorganism that has integrated a bacterial virus (prophage) into its chromosome. In this case, somewhere in the deep mists of time, a bacterial virus infected the vibrio and, unfortunately for the human race, the virus also encoded a gene that controlled not only the synthesis of the deadly toxin but the formation by the vibrio microbe of attachment structures (pili) it used to bind to the epithelial cells of the small intestine it infected. Thus, one gene regulates the expression of both factors required for virulence of *Vibrio cholerae*. There are two main biotypes that have been recognized in pandemics: El Tor and classic. The first El Tor biotype was recognized in a cholera outbreak in Indonesia in 1961 and has spread from a single source in at least three waves over the last sixty years; the single source is the Bay of Bengal, where the ecology and climate is ideal for their propagation. It has caused over five million cases of cholera and over quarter of a million deaths, especially in Africa. This biotype, amazingly enough, contains a protein on its surface that is present on the surfaces of many cells in the body, including red blood cells. It is called the "O" antigen. Thus, the proper name for the biotype is O1 El Tor. How it contributes to pathogenicity is not really understood. However, a genetic variant of the El Tor biotype appeared in Bangladesh in 1992, called the O139 strain, and the composition of the O antigen changed, resulting in the synthesis of a capsule around the strain, which could definitely have a role in pathogenicity by resisting phagocytosis, as other capsulated pathogens do. A number of different chemical properties of the organism also provide us with clues concerning its ability to cause disease. It is highly resistant to alkaline conditions and salt but is very sensitive to acid. Thus, it can survive in highly saline conditions in the ocean, but in order to cause cholera the human body must be infected by tremendously large numbers of organisms (one hundred million to one billion) in order to overcome the acidity of the stomach. However, if for some reason the individual is also consuming an acid-neutralizing drink or pill such as bicarbonate, the number of cholera organisms required for causing disease decreases significantly (as few as 10,000 organisms). Quite remarkable.

3) PATHOGENICITY

As with all pathogens, the disease is due to the secretion of toxins by the ingested organism. However, as described above, a number of factors are involved in assuring a "successful" outcome, such as having sufficient numbers of ingested bacteria (from contaminated water) to minimize against the acidity of the stomach, and not being swept away due to continuing digestion. For this latter purpose, the bacteria must be able to attach themselves to the surface of epithelial cells of the small intestine, which they do via their pili. Here they multiply without damaging most of the cells. Once these "demands" are met, the organism can go about its business of causing the disease. The main offender is a secreted exotoxin (Figure 5.12), a protein composed of two parts, A and B, which is similar to a number of other secreted exotoxins. The B part (which is not toxic) attaches to receptor sites on the epithelial cells. This then allows the A part, which *is* toxic, to penetrate the cell and to carry out its main function, which is to activate an important cellular enzyme called adenylate cyclase. The enzyme converts the high-energy storage compound ATP to a molecule called cyclic AMP. It is cyclic AMP, which is now permanently activated, that reacts with another protein, the "G" protein, which is involved in regulating fluid secretion from the cell. Ordinarily, the G protein is transiently activated and deactivated by the presence or absence of cyclic AMP. However, with the permanent activation of the G protein, massive amounts of fluids, including water, chloride, and other electrolytes, are constantly being secreted across the cell membrane of the epithelial cells. Although the large

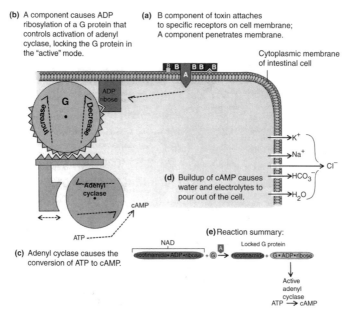

(b) A component causes ADP ribosylation of a G protein that controls activation of adenyl cyclase, locking the G protein in the "active" mode.

(a) B component of toxin attaches to specific receptors on cell membrane; A component penetrates membrane.

Cytoplasmic membrane of intestinal cell

(c) Adenyl cyclase causes the conversion of ATP to cAMP.

(d) Buildup of cAMP causes water and electrolytes to pour out of the cell.

(e) Reaction summary:

Mode of Action of Cholera Toxin As with other A-B toxins, the B portion attaches the toxin to the host cell, and the A portion penetrates the cell and causes toxicity. In this case, the target of the A portion is a G protein responsible for regulating production of cAMP.

FIGURE 5.12 How cholera exotoxin acts on the cell. (See Plate 20)

intestine is not affected by the toxin, it cannot absorb all the fluid, and diarrhea results.

It would not be inappropriate to ask why this is. Why did a nonpathogenic marine microbe gain the capacity (through an infection by a bacterial virus) of producing a toxin that can decimate a human population? Of what possible selective advantage was it for the organism? Perhaps because so many cholera organisms are shed during the course of the disease (over a million per milliliter of fluid), it is a way to ensure continuation of the biotype. Nevertheless, this possibility is just speculation.

Does *V. cholerae* secrete other exotoxins? Decidedly, yes. One of these is a cell-damaging toxin called a "cytolysin," which produces "pores" in the cell membrane of intestinal cells, resulting in the leakage of important metabolic molecules that leads to cell damage or lysis of the cell. Not only that, but after releasing the soluble cytolysin, it can attack cells at a distance, even entering the blood stream to cause further damage. Such pore-forming toxins are secreted by a variety of human pathogens, and a number of investigators (Olson and coworkers) are involved in elucidating the steps involved in the formation of the pores in the cholera organism. As was discussed above with the A and B exotoxin, it is not known how the gene for producing this toxin was acquired and why. Neither is its exact role known in causing cholera.

4) DIAGNOSIS, PREVENTION, AND TREATMENT OF CHOLERA

It is not difficult to determine whether cholera is the cause of an epidemic. The presence of the organism (comma-shaped vibrio) in the diarrhetic excretions of the poor victims provides ample evidence that the disease is present. The more difficult problem is to ascertain how it started and where. One detective story is described in the next part of this chapter section (part 5, titled The Agony of Haiti). There is a vaccine that can provide effective protection for one El Tor biotype (but not the latest one, O139, which arose in Bangladesh) over a short period of time in a high risk situation such as before a trip to an area where cholera might occur or for medical workers in an area where an epidemic is occurring. However, the best protection is measures that provide adequate sewage treatment and a good drinking-water supply, both of which are not usually present in areas where cholera has broken out or where it might break out. Also, it goes without saying that individuals should avoid eating raw food or drinking untested water, among other unhygienic practices, in an infected area.

It is amazing, however, that treatment is very simple and inexpensive and can reduce the mortality rate to less than 1 percent. Since the problem is acute dehydration, rehydration is the answer. Intravenous or oral liquid electrolytes (salts) in pure water are the best therapy. The treatment should be prompt, before damage to vital organs has occurred, although this is not always possible. Sometimes antibiotic therapy with tetracyclins and strepto-mycin can help, but without rehydration this is of little use.

5) THE AGONY OF HAITI

Although there are many outbreaks of cholera all over the world, the one that erupted in the poorest country in the Western Hemisphere, Haiti, in October 2010 is more heartbreaking than others because it came after a huge earthquake early in 2010 that killed perhaps 95,000 people, and it was exacerbated by a hurricane that occurred in November of 2010. One can imagine the chaos and breakdown of sanitation, housing, safe drinking-water supplies, and social services that occurred during these upheavals. Thus, it required not much effort to predict that outbreaks of several kinds of infectious diseases could result, and one, cholera, did. It was caused by the O1 El Tor biotype, but yet it was surprising because no cholera outbreak had been reported in Haiti for over a century. Thus, determining the origin and the means of spread of the disease was necessary to direct a response. Initially it was proposed by numerous sources that the epidemic was directly related to the catastrophic earthquake that had occurred nine months before. However, another possibility was that incoming Nepalese soldiers sent to help restore order in Haiti may have actually been responsible for starting the epidemic because near their camp they emptied waste tanks that leaked into rivers, and most important, there was a cholera outbreak reported in their capital city before they left Nepal. Obviously, it became important to compare cholera organisms from Haiti and South Asia (not Nepal directly, because of political sensitivities). This was carried out by DNA sequencing (genomics; see chapter II, section H), and the organisms were shown to be highly similar. However, the results were challenged and so the controversy is still ongoing. Nevertheless, the fact that the first cases of cholera were found in a tributary of a river near the camp of the soldiers seems to support their unintended role in the epidemic. It is a pity because a good deed of help may have gone awry. Thousands of Haitians have been stricken and died, and still, with more than a million Haitians living in makeshift camps because of the earthquake, vigilance is the key operative term.

6) CONCLUSIONS

In recent outbreaks of cholera in Africa, the mortality rate has increased dramatically, far in excess of the "1 percent" usually recorded. This suggests that existing strains of cholera are evolving toward higher and higher virulence. These strains are probably related to the El Tor biotype, which emerged half a century ago and has spread across the entire planet. Thus, its characterization as a "pretty nasty beast" is well deserved.

G. Influenza: Bird Flu, Swine Flu, and All That Jazz

1) INTRODUCTION

Literally dozens of articles in newspapers around the world, almost daily, have raised an alarm concerning the possibility (or more likely, probability) that the world's population is headed for an outbreak of "bird flu," a viral disease (properly termed Avian influenza) that may have been responsible for one of the most dreaded epidemics (termed a pandemic) ever suffered by the world's population. Called the "Spanish flu," it first appeared in the spring of 1918 and was not exceptionally lethal to those who caught it. However, a second wave, which appeared a few months later, was very lethal and killed between thirty and fifty million people globally. Usually, the mortality rate is very high in the elderly, but in this case, those affected were young to middle-age adults. Why the epidemic was so devastating, why it "jumped" from birds to humans, and whether we are headed for another outbreak, which has been predicted to kill up to 100 million people worldwide, has concerned scientists and officials from many countries. Are these doomsday scenarios realistic or are we in the throes of media hype? Let us provide some answers. First, the twentieth century and the first decade of the twenty-first century have witnessed four flu pandemics, with three occurring in the twentieth century (the last one, in 1968, called the Hong Kong flu) and one in the twenty-first century in 2009 (called the swine flu). None of the four have resulted in the catastrophic death rate seen in 1918. Second, the influenza virus that has caused most of the fear in the past two years (before the swine flu) is an avian strain called H5N1, which infects a variety of domestic poultry, wild birds, and other migratory waterfowl. Literally millions and millions of such birds have been infected and killed since 1997. Yet, although the human toll is mounting slightly, approximately only 150 persons in the Far East and Turkey have caught the disease, with over half the cases being fatal. However, as far as is known, not one infection has resulted from human to human transmission, as is the case with human influenza. Third, this avian strain was first discovered not in Hong Kong in 1997, but in Scotland in 1959. This must mean that literally millions and millions of individuals have come in contact with strain H5N1 for more than fifty years, without any "mutation" that might cause it to become extraordinarily lethal and contagious from person to person. Fourth, nevertheless, although human-to-human transmission has not occurred, that does not mean it cannot occur in the future, and it is prudent to learn as much as is possible about this virus strain and how humans might react to it. One gigantic and remarkable advance in this respect has been the use of genomics to resurrect the exact avian virus strain that was responsible for the deadly 1918 pandemic. How this was accomplished is a marvel in itself, too complex to go into here, but the entire genotype (gene sequence) was determined and yielded some interesting results. For example, it is more lethal to experimental animals than any other human flu virus known, it causes severe inflammation of the lungs (similar to that seen in 1918 victims), and it has the ability to grow in many different cell types.

With this initial introduction, we will now embark on a more detailed study of the influenza virus, its pathogenicity, and how it can mutate to become more virulent and adaptable to different species.

2) THE VIRUS AND PATHOGENICITY

Influenza virus has an unusually complex structure, especially for its genome (genetic material or chromosome), again demonstrating these supposedly "simple" microorganisms are anything but that (Figure 5.13). There are three types of influenza virus—A, B, and C—of which type A is the most common and the one that has a very wide host range, infecting many animals, sea mammals, and birds. It was this group that was responsible for the deadly pandemic of 1918, and a subtype of A (H5N1) is now causing so much concern in birds. The other two types infect only humans and do not cause pandemics.

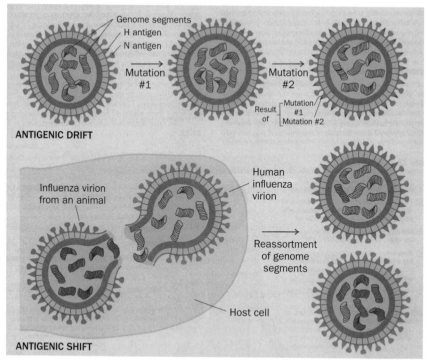

FIGURE 5.13 Influenza virus: Antigenic drift and antigenic shift. With drift, repeated mutations cause gradual change in the antigens composing the hemagglutinin, so that antibody against the original virus becomes progressively less effective. With shift, there is an abrupt, major change in the hemagglutinin antigens because the virus acquires a new genome segment, which in this case codes for hemagglutinin. Changes in neuraminidase could occur by the same mechanism. (See Plate 21)

All three types of virus are similar in structure and in how they replicate, but they differ in proteins that make up their capsid envelope. The shape of the influenza virus is highly variable—sometimes round, sometimes elongated, and sometime bent. Nevertheless, individual virions are surrounded by a lipid-containing capsid envelope, which is derived from the host itself (like the virus HIV, which causes AIDS). Standing out or projecting from the surface are two kinds of spikes essential for attaching to specific host cell receptors. They are made of sugars and proteins (glycoproteins), like so many other attachment organelles of viruses. One is termed hemagglutinin (HA) because it also agglutinates (or clumps) red blood cells, while the other is called neuraminidase (NA). The former enables the virus to bind specific receptors on host epithelial cells (which line the surface of all tissues, including the lungs), while the latter degrades the mucus that is present in the lungs to enable the virus to penetrate to the cell surface. It is interesting that HA can also agglutinate red blood cells, which has been useful in diagnostic procedures since there can be a number of different HA subtypes that arise, as discussed below, which would be important to know prior to developing an appropriate vaccine. Within the capsid envelope there is a matrix protein membrane that protects the inner part of the virus, containing the genetic material or genome. It is the genome of the influenza virus, comprising eight different single-stranded RNA molecules (each one covered by a separate helical coat), that is responsible for the tremendous variability in generating different or new strains of the virus, because such variability lies in the genes that code for HA and NA by processes known as "antigenic drift" and "antigenic shift." In the former, a large number of mutations in the genes that code for HA and NA accumulate within one strain of the virus in a specific geographic area, leading to new strains that can erupt every few years to produce a major but not necessarily severe epidemic. In the latter, a radically new virus strain that codes for new HA and NA proteins emerges when the RNA of different influenza strains is incorporated into the same virion during replication after infection of the same human or animal host cells. This outcome occurs approximately every ten years or so, producing what can be a serious, major epidemic. In effect, the number of possible influenza strains is almost infinite because of antigenic drift and shift. Asia is a major site of antigenic shift and the source of most pandemic strains because there are so many reservoirs of ducks, chickens, and pigs.

This variability is generated during development of the virus, after it has penetrated the cytoplasm of the cell by a process similar to phagocytic engulfment (known as endocytosis) (see Figure 1.7 in chapter I). Host cell metabolism then ceases. Single-stranded viral RNA is released and uses a bound, RNA-dependent polymerase enzyme to synthesize new RNA. However, this RNA is a complement—the (+) strand—of the original (−)-strand RNA chromosome, and this (+) strand then acts as a template to resynthesize many copies of the correct (−)-strand chromosome for formation of progeny virions. In addition, it is the (+) strand that is also used as a template for gene expression via transcription and translation, not the (−) strand, which is why influenza is known as a "minus-strand" RNA virus. Sounds complicated, but that is nothing compared to the complications that arise because the RNA exists as eight separate pieces, each of which is covered as described above. Six of the eight pieces contain a gene that encodes a single protein. The remaining two segments code for two proteins by overlapping genes (in a manner similar to other viruses, such as HIV) (see Figure 5.2 and Table 5.1 in this chapter). It is during the process of new RNA synthesis that mistakes occur in replication, resulting in altered gene sequences (mutations) coding for HA and NA to produce new influenza strains via antigenic drift. All this occurs very rapidly as new nucleoproteins are produced. Within six hours, regions of the host cell membrane become saturated with embedded viral HA and NA proteins, and mature virions start to bud off the host cell enclosed by this structurally altered cell-membrane envelope. They then spread to nearby cells in the lung, including those cells that secrete the protective mucus in the alveoli, which are infected and die very quickly. This impairs a major nonspecific defense system of the body, allowing secondary infections (such as several types of pneumonia) to develop as well. In fact, it was calculated that over 20% of the deaths occurring during the deadly 1918 pandemic were due to these secondary pneumonia infections. Nevertheless, the immune system is working overtime to kill infected cells, and inflammatory factors (cytokines) are released to aid the process, although such inflammation produces the typical symptoms of flu. Most people who acquire flu are cured, but still there are minorities of the elderly, children, pregnant women, or already sick people who can succumb. Because the infection is so widespread and can occur every year, the total number of deaths is quite high. An estimated 10,000 to 30,000 deaths occur from the human strains each year in the United States alone.

The latest influenza virus concern (2009) arose from a subtype of influenza virus A, called H1N1. Initially recognized in Mexico, it spread worldwide, causing the World Health Organization (WHO) to label it a pandemic. Known commonly as the "swine flu" because half of its genetic makeup is derived from swine, this virus represented a remarkable example of "antigenic shift" in which the remaining half of its genetic elements were derived from human and avian viruses. Of interest is that, like during the deadly 1918 pandemic, the elderly population was more resistant than younger adults and children, probably because they were exposed to similar viruses in their youth. It is most likely that because of the relative mildness of the infection, the pandemic ran its course relatively quickly, and the WHO declared it over in one year. A very important issue relating to public policy was that millions of dollars were appropriated by many countries for various purposes related to treatment facilities, health care, and research, and millions of dollars more were spent on preparing millions of doses of vaccine. As it turned out, most of these initiatives were not used and thus could have been considered "wasted." But were they? It cannot be determined beforehand whether an outbreak of an infectious disease such as influenza will continue, and how severe it could become. For example, a mutation may have occurred in the H1N1 virus, rendering it more deadly. Thus, it was prudent to err on the side of caution and to be prepared for any eventuality. One positive aspect of the H1N1 pandemic was the cooperation that arose in the "international medical community," which can be revitalized quickly if required again.

3) SPREAD, PREVENTION, AND TREATMENT

Since viral HA and NA antigens from new flu strains appear almost yearly, this will ensure that susceptible individuals will always be present when the disease strikes, usually in the late fall and winter. Infection occurs primarily through inhalation of airborne viruses expelled by sneezing or coughing from other infected individuals, but the disease is also easily spread by self-contamination, such as by touching one's mouth or nose with contaminated fingers, which is why washing or personal hygiene is so important in preventing its spread. Infected individuals are contagious as early as one day after visible signs of the disease appear, and they remain that way for at least a week. Amazingly enough, carriers of the disease who exhibit no symptoms also exist. Early diagnosis is essential for the production of the right vaccine, and symptoms are easily spotted by physicians, although a number of more accurate laboratory tests are required to distinguish which strain of the flu is the culprit. Antiviral therapy, either by drugs or by vaccines, can be used for treatment. In the latter case, the actual virus strain (which is first cultured in eggs and then inactivated) or its specific hemagglutinin antigen can be used to prepare the vaccine. The vaccines are between 60 and 90% effective, which is vital in helping susceptible individuals survive. There are at present four drugs that have been approved to treat flu. They act either to prevent uncoating of the virus, to inhibit the action of neuraminidase, or to block the release of new viruses from infected cells. They must be taken during the first forty-eight hours to be effective, and the virus can develop resistance to them, as shown by the 2005–2006 strain, which is resistant to two of the four drugs. Although hundreds of millions of dollars are spent annually on pain relievers and antihistamines to relieve the symptoms of flu, aspirin and its derivatives should not be among them because of an increased risk of Reye's syndrome, a fatal syndrome characterized by liver and brain damage, mostly of children with fever. Another rare complication is that of Guillain-Barre syndrome, which occurs rarely in vaccinated individuals. It is characterized by severe paralysis, but most people recover completely. In fact, one of the most famous cases was that of the author Joseph Heller, who wrote the classic *Catch 22*. Unfortunately, it took him years to recover, which is why pharmaceutical companies that develop vaccines are becoming fewer and fewer due to the possibility of lawsuits from side effects. It should not be that way! The federal government should ensure that such companies are covered, since vaccines are one of the mainstays of prevention for so many infectious diseases. This is especially true for the latest scare of a pandemic from the H5N1 strain of bird flu, which still could occur. A number of countries, including the United States, France, and Russia, are experimenting with a prototype of a pandemic flu vaccine against this strain, which shows promise. It is impossible to predict whether a bird flu pandemic will occur in the future, and if it does, it may not be the exact same H5N1 strain because of antigenic shift or drift. Therefore, very quick action must be taken to determine what strain is involved, so that vaccine production can begin immediately. Fortunately, thus far there has been little if any further spread of this virus. Instead, most of the international medical community's efforts were directed to combating the 2009 H1N1 (swine flu) pandemic virus, which ended quickly after one year, as discussed above. Nevertheless, due to the fact that many children or young adults, pregnant women, immune-compromised individuals, and the elderly may be at more risk, depending upon the strain of the flu virus, a stockpile of vaccine should always remain for a time even in developed countries, which has not always been the case. Unfortunately, pediatric vaccination still remains a problem, and the fact that so many people (infected or not) will flood doctors' offices and hospitals suggests that a severe strain on such medical facilities can occur. This chaos has been true for all such pandemics, even those that are seasonal.

4) CONCLUSION

In conclusion, influenza is a serious and deadly viral disease for which we always must be prepared. However, whether we should concentrate primarily on the possibility of a bird flu pandemic or ensure that the human influenza outbreaks we face every year are rigorously understood and treated is a matter for debate. Yet, it seems obvious that the latter is more important, given the number of cases that emerge. As for bird flu, we have time and the great technologies of modern science to prepare ourselves should it strike.

6

Biofilms: City of Microbes and their Role in Pathogenicity

A. Introduction

Of the many shocks to microbiologists studying how microorganisms actually live in nature, and, as important, how they cause infectious diseases, the perception that bacteria have a unicellular lifestyle under most environmental conditions has been seriously challenged. Yet, since their discovery, that is how they have been traditionally studied and exploited. It is certainly the case that many microbial phenomena, including their pathogenicity, have been elucidated by studying such a unicellular lifestyle. Nevertheless, for a number of years it has been known that most microorganisms live in highly structured communities in nature. That's right! Such communities come complete with a highly complex channeling network, a means of communication, cooperative functions, and protection against outside insults such as antibiotics and drugs. In addition, these communities can comprise many different species, all acting to protect or ensure that the community is working properly. Such "social" organizations have been labeled "biofilms." Hence, although bacteria can exist independently, they mostly congregate or aggregate into a community in many different environments, including the human and animal body. It is there that biofilms can have a dramatic and profound effect on the cause and outcome of a specific infection. Yet, there are "good" biofilms, such as those that protect an internal human niche in the gastrointestinal tract or oral cavity (mouth) from harmful biofilms. This is an enormous field that has just come into great prominence, especially, as stated above, because of the role of these biofilms in maintaining or causing chronic infections. Thus, we will explore how they form, their properties, and their remarkable activities in this "city of microbes."

B. Biofilms and Infectious Diseases

The first detailed report of the structural nature of biofilms was published in 1991 by three Canadian scientists, J. R. Lawrence, D. Caldwell, and J. W. Coster-ton. Their important contribution was to use a different kind of microscope to view these large communities, instead of an ordinary light microscope. The instrument is called a confocal microscope, which can scan through planes of the biofilm in depth, by a technique called laser scanning. In this way, the bacteria were shown to group themselves in small "enclaves," with all the groups surrounded by a gluelike polysaccharide or other substance that trapped small particles and absorbed water. It is this glue that holds the biofilm together and enhances the formation of the complex structure within it, which consists basically of channels to allow water and nutrients to flow to various parts of the microbial enclaves while at the same time removing end (waste) products of metabolism. However, not all the microbial groups receive the same level of nutrients. Those at the edge of the biofilm do, but those in the deeper parts do not and must somehow absorb nutrients as best they can. Actually, the levels of nutrients are still sufficient to allow them to metabolize but not to multiply as quickly as those nearer the edge. Oxygen is an important player in the metabolism of the cells in the biofilm because it will determine the energy levels present and whether the bacteria can multiply or not. Thus, it has been determined that oxygen levels can vary greatly within the biofilm and control how the various microbial groups respond metabolically. Each biofilm may be huge in comparison to the size of a colony of free-living bacteria, ranging from hundreds of microns to almost a thousand microns in depth. Such a range is astonishing when one considers that a micron is one millionth of a meter, and one average bacterial cell is between 0.3 and 0.5 of a micron.

There are generally four to five steps involved in the formation and expansion of a biofilm (Figure 6.1). The first is that free-living bacteria (called planktonic cells) make contact with a surface on which they will attach. They then migrate toward each other, using their "organelles of motion," the flagella and pili (long appendages that thrust outward from many bacteria to enable them to stick to the surface). Once the individual cells make contact, they become immobilized. Thus, some signal is expressed to inhibit further activity by the flagella. A microcolony is soon formed. The second step is that the microcolony starts to excrete the gluelike polysaccharide or other substance to contain the budding biofilm and to allow the cells within to grow and start forming a complex structure. The third step consists of the actual formation of the biofilm structure, which includes the formation of channels, the organization of the various microcolonies at various sites in the biofilm that are best suited for their needs, and other aspects of their activities, such as the secretion of "communication" molecules that enable all these activities to occur. The fourth step involves either the continued development of the biofilm or

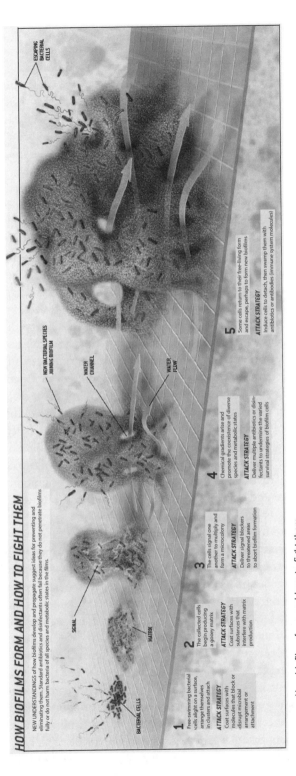

HOW BIOFILMS FORM AND HOW TO FIGHT THEM

NEW UNDERSTANDINGS of how biofilms develop and propagate suggest ideas for preventing and eliminating them. Standard antibiotics and disinfectants often fail because they do not penetrate biofilms fully or do not harm bacteria of all species and metabolic states in the films.

ESCAPING BACTERIAL CELLS

NEW BACTERIAL SPECIES JOINING BIOFILM

WATER CHANNEL

WATER FLOW

SIGNAL

MATRIX

BACTERIAL CELLS

1
Free-swimming bacterial cells alight on a surface, arrange themselves in clusters and attach

ATTACK STRATEGY
Coat surfaces with molecules that block or disrupt microbial arrangement or attachment

2
The collected cells begin producing a gooey matrix

ATTACK STRATEGY
Coat surfaces with substances that interfere with matrix production

3
The cells signal one another to multiply and form a microcolony

ATTACK STRATEGY
Deliver signal blockers to threatened areas to abort biofilm formation

4
Chemical gradients arise and promote the coexistence of diverse species and metabolic states

ATTACK STRATEGY
Deliver multiple antibiotics or disinfectant to undermine the varied survival strategies of biofilm cells

5
Some cells return to their free-living form and escape, perhaps to form new biofilms

ATTACK STRATEGY
Induce cells to detach, then swamp them with antibiotics or antibodies (immune system molecules)

FIGURE 6.1 How biofilms form and how to fight them.

its actual dissolution, depending on outside conditions. However, the entire biofilm will not be degraded at once. Cells are free to leave or join the biofilm, and, indeed, some cells will actually undergo self-destruction to provide nutrients to the remaining biofilm, depending on the availability of outside nutrients. One can imagine that many different genes are expressed in the development of the biofilm itself; this development differs from gene expression by free-living planktonic cells. These include genes that express products to suppress flagella movement, secrete the exopolysaccharide protective mass, and control the expression of "communication" or sensing molecules (among many others). This latter phenomenon has been termed "quorum sensing"; these genes consist of small molecules that diffuse away from cells in one microcolony to those of another (or vice versa) that somehow signal the latter to act in a certain way, such as to redistribute themselves to another part of the biofilm, to alter protein expression, to stimulate the transfer of genetic traits, or to start forming channels by secreting certain lipids that act as biosurfactants (microdetergents) to prevent water from penetrating the cells. How the sensing molecules control these reactions is still largely unknown, but they have been identified both in natural and cultured biofilms. One of them (termed acyl HSL) has shown to be involved in a number of the above activities. Mutants that do not produce these quorum sensors cannot form a biofilm. Another very interesting property of biofilms is the presence of "persistor" cells. These consist of slow-growing cells that resist many antimicrobial agents used during attempts to destroy the biofilm in infected hosts. It is not that these cells are mutants genetically resistant to a particular antibiotic or drug, but they simply are able to survive better under existing conditions, perhaps because it is difficult for the drug to penetrate the sites where they are present. Thus, when other sensitive cells are destroyed by the drug or antibiotic, the biofilm can be reformed and become even more resistant because it will be made up mostly of persistor cells.

Biofilms are involved in many aspects of pathogenesis. It is impossible to list them all, but the most common biofilm infection (mainly by staphylococci) occurs after implants of various devices such as prosthetic valves, which are the leading cause of heart infections in patients who have undergone heart valve replacement. Mortality can be as high as 70%. Also, millions of catheters are inserted into patients every year, which can lead to the formation of biofilms, even if the insertions were done carefully. The immune state of the individual is important as to whether the biofilm will develop or not. Contact lenses are another source of contamination that can lead to biofilm development. Chronic infections caused by formation of biofilms containing one of the most opportunistic pathogens known (*Pseudomonas aeruginosa*) have been of great concern in patients suffering from cystic fibrosis. Other common chronic infections by other biofilm formers (streptococci) include those of the ear (otitis), teeth (periodontitis), and gums (gingivitis). The main reason for these problems lies, as we pointed out above, in the fact that biofilms are resistant to many adverse effects of stress, such as accumulation of toxic waste products within the cell, and to drug chemotherapy by virtue of their protective exopolysaccharide matrix, persistor cells, development of resistant mutants, etc. Nevertheless, a great deal of additional research is required to determine how the biofilms develop and sometimes remain for decades in such chronic infections, and how they cause disease in humans.

7

Biological Terrorism: Myths and Realities

A. Introduction

A significant number of years have gone by since October 18, 2001, when the first bioterror attack with anthrax spores jarred not only the people of the United States but most of the rest of the world's population as well. Coming so close on the heels of the 9/11 terror attacks by Muslim extremists, it seemed that our nation was on the verge of being assaulted on many fronts and (as many of us thought) that we were facing an enemy as evil as the Nazis in World War II, and in some ways more fanatical. Of course, the number of lives lost to anthrax was minute compared to the horror of 9/11, but the impact—the fear factor—was just as great and perhaps even greater. Fortunately, with the passage of time, we can look back at this double blow to our "solar plexus" as a nation and reflect on how far we have come, how much further we have to go, and the absolute necessity to place bioterror agents into perspective in comparison to other types of terror attacks (with chemicals and explosives, for example).

Soon after the anthrax attack, a number of microbiologists lectured and wrote articles concerning the pathogen itself, to try to assuage the public by describing what anthrax was and how it infected people. Unfortunately, the media were instrumental in spreading unreasonable fear and panic before they had any solid information. Subsequent to the attack, there was concern for those postal workers who handled the contaminated letters that were sent to members of Congress and to television news outlets, and they were given appropriate antibiotics as a precaution (see below).

Nevertheless, of the probable hundreds and perhaps thousands of people exposed to anthrax spores (the form of the bacterium that is spread in the air), only eleven cases of the worst and most fatal type of anthrax (called inhalation or respiratory anthrax) were detected, and of those victims, six were

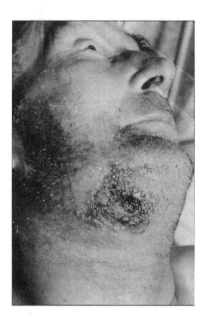

FIGURE 7.1 Cutaneous anthrax. A blackened ulcer at the site of infection.

saved by aggressive treatment, too complex to describe here. The other types include the most common forms of anthrax: "cutaneous" (a skin infection; see Figure 7.1) and "gastrointestinal." Also, approximately only fifty individuals (that we know of) tested positive for anthrax exposure. As a famous president (Franklin D. Roosevelt) stated in one of his memorable speeches about the economic depression, "The only thing we have to fear is fear itself."

In the case of anthrax, that is still largely true. Except under very difficult circumstances (such as disgorging spores over a city, from a low-flying plane), anthrax is not a good bioterror weapon for a number of reasons. It is, as one eminent scientist stated, "a weapon of mass hysteria and not mass destruction." It cannot be spread from person to person, and it has to be prepared carefully by growing it in suitable nutrient solutions to permit spore formation, followed by grinding the mass of spores into very small particles (with silica), which many times can inactivate the anthrax bacterium itself. The terrorists would have to have access to a relatively sophisticated laboratory to create the right particle size, which is why the FBI thought it came from one of our own laboratories that study anthrax. Thus, it seemed that the spore powder that was mailed did not represent a diabolic advance in bioweapon technology, but a routine preparation that required special laboratory facilities.

Other important reasons for why anthrax is a relatively poor choice as a bioweapon include treatment. Unlike viruses, anthrax can be treated successfully with antibiotics, especially during early stages of the disease, which is why diagnostic techniques are very important to develop. Speed of analysis is the key for which treatment to use. Of course, the terrorists could have developed an anthrax bacterium that was resistant to antibiotics (they did not), but in many cases, such resistance leads to defective organisms, which cannot produce spores. A very potent antibiotic, Ciprofloxacin, was first used, which may have been a mistake because it had just been approved as an antibiotic, has a number of side effects, is expensive, and could lead to resistance if not taken continuously. Several other widely available and less expensive antibiotics were as effective, including that old standby penicillin and various tetracyclins. However, one important problem is that once the organism becomes established in the body, it secretes potent toxins that are not susceptible to any antibiotic. The only effective treatment in this scenario would be to use the power of vaccines, which would inactivate the toxins by immune reactions with antibodies, proteins that float around the circulatory system that complex with foreign substances to inactivate them. Unfortunately, at present there is only one source for such a vaccine; namely, the military personnel who have been immunized against the toxins. None of the civilian population has been so immunized. Nevertheless, it is possible to use the technique of "passive immunity," where a small amount of the blood fraction (called the serum, where the antibodies exist) of the more than 100,000 armed-forces personnel who were immunized can be removed and then injected into those victims who have the dreaded form of inhalation anthrax. So, not all is hopeless, by any means. It takes knowledge and effort, of which we have a great abundance.

B. Historical Perspective

There is no "discipline" or field of study called "bioterrorism." It represents a general phrase that encompasses an emerging threat to civilization, and it brings together experts from a variety of scientific and public disciplines, including engineers, microbiologists (and their associated disciplines such as biochemistry and genetics), physicians, epidemiologists, law enforcement and other governmental agencies, and "nonscientific" individuals such as sociologists and historians. Nevertheless, since for the most part the capability of pathogenic bacteria and viruses (or their toxic products) to cause disease makes them the "best" potential agents for biological warfare, it is certain that microbiologists stand at the center of this vortex. In addition, most microbiologists view bioterror research as a continuum of a long-standing effort into the study of emerging and reemerging diseases, which represents a natural evolution between humanity and the much-greater array of microbes. Bioterrorism is part of this process, albeit a deliberate one. In other words, this is not something new but is something familiar, something in which our capabilities are considerable.

However, in general, almost any organism can be used as a bioweapon, and historically, the onslaught goes back even to antiquity, where rotting corpses were hurled over the defenses of fortresses to spread disease. Much closer to our own pre-revolutionary era, when European settlers first came to the Americas, they gave Native Americans blankets as gifts, many of which were contaminated by smallpox virus, a deadly bioterror agent. Native Americans were not immune to smallpox, and many of them perished. I am convinced, however, that this was not intentional, since it was unknown how the disease was caused, much less by an ultramicroscopic, invisible entity. Later on, during World War II, it was commonly suspected that Japan dropped millions of fleas infected with bubonic plague over a number of Chinese cities, and both the Japanese and Nazis experimented with live subjects in efforts to "improve" their deadly agents. Despite the horror of these experiments, the former Soviet Union and other nations, including the United States, Japan, Germany, and, later on, Iraq, China, and probably North Korea, developed or tried to develop biological warfare weapons for anthrax and other agents of mass destruction. Ample evidence exists for many accidents occurring during these developments, such as the release of anthrax spores from a test facility in the former Soviet Union in the 1980s, which resulted in the deaths of many animals and perhaps eighty people. Nevertheless, there is no limitation as to the types of organisms besides bacterial and viral pathogens that can be used as bioterror weapons. Higher parasites are also available, such as the eggs from parasitic roundworms, which were used to infect a number of university students in Montreal in 1970. In other words, it makes sense when considering bioterrorism to include many different types of organisms and their products, so as not to be restricted within a box of "popular" bioterror agents.

As with all catastrophic events, however, the anthrax attack did stimulate an incredible amount of important and useful work. It transformed the priorities of the American government as well as those of the public and scientific communities. There was a remarkable response from scientists around the world who wanted to cooperate with our scientists from governmental agencies, such as the National Institutes of Health, to elucidate how anthrax and other potential bioterror agents could be diagnosed and treated if they were used. It is almost macabre to think that such was the intended aim of the individual who sent the infected letters. Sounds bizarre, I know, but he or she must have recognized that the agent could not kill many people but no doubt would cause a massive response to many aspects of fighting bioterrorism. And as such it did.

C. Bioterrorism Today: State of the Art and Preparedness

Even before the anthrax attack in 2001, a congressional initiative in 1999 began upgrading our public health capabilities to counteract a potential bioterror onslaught. A lead agency, the Centers for Disease Control and Prevention (CDC) in Atlanta, was designated as the primary agency to coordinate all activities related to bioterrorism. Many aspects of concern were considered, including planning, surveillance, diagnostics, therapy, law enforcement, stockpiling of drugs and vaccines, and, perhaps the most important consideration, which pathogens (bacteria and viruses) should be given the highest priority in terms of their danger to humanity. These are the dry facts. Despite such important considerations, not much was implemented until the attack itself. It appeared as if all the discussions had gone to naught and that it required a catastrophe to galvanize the scientific and governmental communities to act more quickly (as has been the case so often in history, such as in World War II, which led to the development of the first antibiotic penicillin). There are still huge gaps in preparedness, as I will detail below, but many important initiatives were implemented as well.

One of the first assessments involved, as stated above, was which biological agents to consider, and for whom. Originally, military concerns or which agents to use to incapacitate soldiers were of prime concern. However, it became quickly obvious that terrorists were also interested, in fact more interested, in harming civilians, such as when Saddam Hussein ordered the murder of thousands of Kurds with poison gas in the 1980s. It became clear that civilian populations have different criteria for evaluation of bioterror agents than does the military, such as a wider age distribution and different health conditions in the former. Civilians are a much more diverse group than the military and much more vulnerable to, for example, food or waterborne bioterror agents. Thus, law enforcement and other agencies needed to be more vigilant in protecting food and water supplies. From considerations such as these, two broad guidelines that had already been laid out in 1999 by infectious-disease and other experts were quickly publicized after the anthrax attack; these guidelines serve until the present as the best approach to select which biological agents and which type of preparedness issues to consider. Of course, as with every "list" or guideline, there is the danger or difficulty of remaining static and not changing such considerations when faced with changing conditions. Bacteria and viruses never remain the same and are always evolving into new and perhaps more-dangerous pathogens (not to mention terrorists attempting to hasten and "improve" such disease-causing capabilities). Nevertheless, it is a starting point and in my opinion a good and comprehensive one.

The first guideline deals with critical agent categories for public health preparedness, which are divided into three classes (categories A–C). Category A agents have the greatest potential for mass destruction and require the greatest preparedness capabilities, such as maintaining a stockpile of drugs and rapid methods to diagnose them. These are the agents that have the greatest potential for lethality, spread, and generating fear in the civilian population. They include five powerful bacterial and viral pathogens, including smallpox (virus), anthrax (bacterial), bubonic or sylvatic (spread by aerosol) plague (bacterial), botulism toxin (poison produced by a bacterium), tularemia (causing debilitating effects in humans; bacterial), and hemorrhagic fevers (viral, such as Ebola, Marburg, and Lassa). There are a number of problems with this list, including the fact that I dismissed anthrax as a truly serious biological danger (as described in the first section of this chapter). Nevertheless, it is precisely because it has been used as a weapon and has generated great fear and panic that it probably was included in category A. In addition, there are a relatively large number of other diseases that could have been included in this category because they display the same indicators as the ones chosen. However, it probably would have required too-many resources to deal with them in a high-priority category. Category B agents also have a strong potential for illness and its spread, but according to the current thinking they cause less severe symptoms, although this is debatable for some of them. I think the primary reason for this category is that the public is not as aware of them as those in category A, although this too is debatable. I will not list all the agents, but they include exotic diseases such as brucellosis and glanders (both animal diseases that can spread to man); Q fever, typhus, and encephalitis (different diseases that are caused by parasites that lie midway between viruses and bacteria, known as rickettsia); cholera; and typhoid. These latter two diseases (waterborne and food centered, respectively), caused by bacteria, should, in my strong view, be placed in category A because they are well known, have a great fear factor, and can be spread easily. Finally, category C agents are not thought to represent a high threat now, but they could become one as more knowledge is gained through research. It is interesting that both SARS (severe acute respiratory syndrome) and flu (influenza virus) have not been included in any list, primarily because they would be exceedingly difficult to control, and if restrictions were placed on where and how they could be studied, it could lead to a stifling of research.

The second broad guideline concerns criteria for evaluating the potential bioterror agents, which led to the assignment of which agents to place in the three categories described above. There were six different factors considered, including (1) the degree of threat, (2) mortality, (3) ease with which the agent is spread, (4) ease with which the agent is spread between people, (5) public perception (fear factor), and (6) ease or difficulty of preparation. Such considerations resulted in category A agents having the highest number of "positive" rankings. For example, smallpox would rank higher than Q fever because of its greater untreated lethality, as well as its greater spread potential. The same would hold true for plague because of its greater mortality rates. One important criterion for any agent in any category is the ease of preparing and spreading them. This consideration seems to be the weakest link, in my view, for would-be terrorists. Generating the "right" particle size as well as the right culture conditions requires special knowledge about handling aerosols, including physical knowledge of the right viscosity (thickness) and temperature of the fluid or powder in which the agent is carried. All these factors are necessary to maintain its virulence, and this is especially true for viruses. Yet, despite all these potential problems, the fervor and deviousness of terrorists may, under the right circumstances, circumvent them. It is the speed of travel that could be the primary culprit. A determined terrorist who is not averse to committing suicide (albeit in a horrible way) could be infected and, before symptoms develop, travel to a foreign destination such as any big city, where he could develop the disease and infect many innocent people before succumbing. This may be an unlikely scenario, but not so different from crashing an airliner into the twin towers of the World Trade Center on September 11, 2001.

In facing the challenges of bioterrorism, the National Institutes of Health in 2003 put forth a major plan for biodefense research, which balanced basic and applied research and would total over 1.7 billion dollars, if implemented. Proposals included construction of high-containment laboratories at various research centers, increasing basic research on bioterror agents, expanding training programs, testing of new drugs and vaccines, establishing repositories for such drugs and vaccines, expanding clinical trials of drugs and vaccines, and engaging industry in the overall effort. In the latter activity, a new program called the Project Bioshield Act was passed by the Congress and signed by the then president George W. Bush in 2004. It is a ten-year, 5.6-billion-dollar project designed to give financial assurances to biotech and pharmaceutical companies that are somewhat nervous about spending their funds on products with a limited market. It guarantees that any new product for biodefense that a company develops will be bought by the federal government, and it decreases the time for approving the product. However, not only are such firms being solicited, but research is already underway at a number of governmental facilities, and there is a heightened degree of cooperation between such facilities and those in other countries. Thus, an effective vaccine against two of the most insidious bioterror threats, Ebola and Marburg viruses, has recently been developed by scientists from the Public Health Agency in Canada and the US Army Medical Research Institute in Maryland. Not only were these frightening diseases almost 100% fatal in outbreaks in Africa, but, as reported recently in the *New York Times*, a Russian defector in the 1990s claimed that the Soviets had stockpiled Marburg virus and were able to process it for use in missiles. Another government laboratory, Lawrence Livermore Labs, in California, which used to be involved in nuclear-weapons research, changed after 9/11. As reported in the *Wall Street Journal*, they are busy designing and testing a novel "pathogen detection system." Literally a portable laboratory the size of a small refrigerator, it can rapidly test for over ninety separate pathogens, including anthrax and plague. The overall plan is ideal, but as with all such plans, the realities are another problem. For example, few communities want a high-containment laboratory facility in their "neighborhood." Accidents have happened and the fear for an escape of a bioterror agent (although unlikely) is still a fear. Nevertheless, the new awareness has resulted in concrete steps to minimize the fear and panic of a possible attack. For example, in 2004, a white powder was discovered in the Senate majority leader's mailroom. Analysis showed that the powder contained ricin, an extremely potent toxin extracted from castor beans that was used in international terrorism in the 1970s, when a Hungarian diplomat was stabbed (and subsequently died) by an umbrella impregnated with the toxin. Although not a bacterial or viral bioterror agent, it is an example of thinking about such agents "outside the box." Unlike the anthrax scare, however, this incident was managed very well due to better preparedness since 2001. No one was harmed and there was only a short temporary closing of the Senate office building.

D. Conclusions

One of the most serious problems our nation faces with respect to bioterror preparedness lies with the bureaucracy both of the federal and state governments, but largely with the states. Despite massive defense spending, many efforts are lagging in the states. This is where the bottleneck lies. A nonpartisan organization (Trust for America's Health) evaluated ten preparedness indicators in public health awareness of bioterrorism. Although all fifty states had plans approved by the CDC in Atlanta, twenty-six states failed to spend their allotted bioterror funds, thirty-nine states did not make state-specific information about specific diseases available to the general public, and forty-eight states did not have enough trained staff to receive and distribute supplies and medicine from a national repository. In all, only four states met most of the recommendations approved by the nonpartisan organization mentioned above. Such low compliance rates were attributed to state budget cuts and to the various bureaucracies in the state governments themselves, where there were major disagreements between local health agencies in the capital and in the other cities and towns of the state. Clearly, if our nation is to meet the horror of a bioterror attack, all the parts of the state and federal government have to cooperate and do much more than they are doing now. There is a terrible danger, and we would be absolutely delinquent in letting these problems continue to fester.

GLOSSARY

This glossary includes famous and not-so-famous individuals who have contributed significantly in opening our world to the "infectious microbe." Not all of them were scientists, especially during the early years of endeavor. They range from simple monks, craftsmen who ground glass into lenses, and naturalists between the sixteenth and nineteenth centuries; to chemists, physicians, early geneticists and cell biologists, pathologists, and microbiologists interested in the causes of diseases between the late eighteenth and nineteenth centuries; and finally, to the myriad of specialists of the modern era in the fields of microbiology, molecular biology, biochemistry, genetics, immunology, and biophysics between the twentieth century and the present. A significant number of the scientists listed have won the Nobel Prize for their research in microbiology or immunology.

A. Scientists

Avery, O. Codiscoverer with C. Macleod and M. McCarty of transformation of genetic traits by DNA, the first demonstration that the chemical DNA carries genetic information (1944).

Bang, B. L. Discovered organism that causes brucellosis (undulant fever) (1904).

Beadle, G. Codiscoverer with E. Tatum of how genes functioned by controlling the synthesis of specific enzymes. Coined the "one-gene, one-enzyme" hypothesis (1941). Won Nobel Prize in 1958.

Beijerinck, M. W. Codiscoverer with D. Iwanowski of the existence of viruses (1898).

Caldwell, D. (see Costerton, J. W.)

Calmette, A. Developed (along with C. Guerin) a vaccine called "BCG" (Bacillus Calmette-Guerin) by using a weakened or attenuated strain of a closely related tuberculosis (TB) organism that infects cattle. Used in Europe and Africa but not the United States.

Costerton, J. W. Codiscoverer with D. Caldwell and J. R. Lawrence of the first detailed characterization of biofilms (city of microbes) (1991).

Crick, F. C. Codiscoverer with J. D. Watson of double-helix structure of DNA (1953). Won Nobel Prize in 1962.

Ehrenberg, C. G. von. Developed first "classification" of microorganisms (1838).

Ehrlich, P. Searched for and developed the first chemotherapeutic agent ("salvosan") to treat syphilis (1897). Won Nobel Prize in 1908.

Falkow, S. Outstanding medical microbiologist who recognized that most virulence factors are common to most pathogens.

Fleischmann, R. D. Demonstrated that laboratory cultivation of TB strains weakened the virulence of TB organisms compared to those freshly isolated strains (2005).

Fracastorius, G. Earliest suggestion that a "contagum virum" (bad air) was responsible for spreading disease (1540).

Francis, E. Discovered organism that causes tularemia (rabbit fever) (1922).

Frankel, A. Discovered the organism that causes pneumonia (1886).

Griffith, F. Detected a factor from heat-killed pneumococci that "transformed" nonvirulent pneumococcal mutants to virulent ones in mice, capable of causing pneumonia (1928). This phenomenon was reinvestigated by Avery, MacLeod, and McCarty in 1944 to demonstrate that the factor was DNA.

Guerin, C. See Calmette, A.

Houghton, J. M. Proposed (along with T. Wang) that long-term inflammation of the stomach epithelium cells by *Helicobacter pylori*, the cause of ulcers, attracts stem cells from the bone marrow, which develop into cancer cells due to the chronic inflammation (2005).

Iwanowski, D. Codiscoverer (with M. Beijerinck) of the existence of viruses (1898).

Jacob, F. Outstanding microbial geneticist who along with A. Lwoff, J. Monod, and E. Wollman proposed the "operon" model for genetic control of gene expression. Jacob and Monod won the Nobel Prize in 1965.

Jenner, E. First use of vaccination to treat disease through the application of attenuated (weakened) viruses that caused smallpox and rabies (1796).

Karström, H. Discovered the phenomenon of "adaptive" enzyme formation, in which enzymes are activated to metabolize their specific substrates when they are present (1937).

Kitasato, S. Discovered organism that causes tetanus (1889) and simultaneously with Yersin, bubonic plague (1894).

Klebs, E. Discovered the organism that causes diphtheria (1883).

Koch, R. One of the founding fathers of medical microbiology, who engaged in extensive research on tuberculosis and cholera and described necessary methods for studying the germ theory of disease (Koch's postulates) (1876). Won Nobel Prize in 1905.

Lancefield, R. First characterized and separated streptococci into four main groups depending on immunological reactions to their surface antigens (1935).

Lawrence, J. R. See Costerton, J. W.

Lederberg, J. Brilliant microbiologist who discovered recombinant processes in microorganisms, including conjugation and transduction (1952). Won the Nobel Prize in 1958.

Leunk, R. Detection of antibody against *Helicobacter pylori* toxin in individuals suffering from ulcers but not in normal individuals, suggesting that the toxin is produced in vivo and that it could contribute to the pathology of the disease (1990).

Lwoff, A. See Jacob, F.

MacLeod, C. See Avery, O.

Marshall, B. J. Codiscoverer with J. R. Warren that ulcers were caused by the bacterium *Helicobacter pylori* (1983). Won the Nobel Prize in 2005.

McCarty, M. See Avery, O.

Meischer, F. Discovered the chemical DNA (1869).

Monod, J. See Jacob, F.

Muller, O. First revealed structural details within microorganisms (1786).

Nathanson, N. Respected epidemiologist who first recognized that emerging diseases are influenced by human activities that fall into three general societal categories; namely, rapid transportation, explosive growth of human populations, and severe upsets in the environment (1990s).

Olson, R. Elucidating structural details of the unusual pore forming toxin of cholera.

Pasteur, L. One of the founding fathers of medical microbiology, who proposed the first germ theory for disease, developed a method (pasteurization, 1864) that destroyed most pathogens in foods that could not be boiled, disproved the theory of spontaneous generation (in which live organisms arose from dead organic material), and used attenuated (weakened) organisms to prepare effective vaccines against rabies and anthrax (1860–1870).

Plenciz, M. A. von. First enunciated the idea that diseases are caused by "minute organisms" floating in the air (1762).

Prowazek, S. Codiscovered with H. Ricketts the small organism that causes typhus (1905).

Ricketts, H. Discovered with S. Prowazek the small organism that causes typhus (1905).

Rous, P. Discovered that certain viruses could cause cancer (Rous sarcoma) in chickens (1913).

Salk, J. Virologist who developed the first vaccine against polio, by using three different inactivated polio virus strains (1955).

Schlievert, P. First characterization of toxins that act as superantigens (1982).

Tatum, E. See Beadle, G.

Trucksis, O. M. Studies tuberculosis in goldfish, a model system that mimics many of the symptoms of human TB and at a faster rate, resulting in the detection of new virulence genes (2005).

van Leeuwenhoek, A. Constructed the first microscope and was the first to view bacteria, algae, and other microscopic forms (1674).

Waksman, S. Discovered streptomycin, the first useful antibiotic to treat tuberculosis. Won the Nobel Prize in 1952.

Wang, T. See Houghton, J. M.

Warren, J. R. See Marshall, B. J.

Watson, J. See Crick, F. C.

Wechselbaum, A. Discovered the organism that causes most of the cases of meningitis (1887).

Wollman, E. See Jacob, F.

Yersin, A. Simultaneously with S. Kitasato, discovered the organism that causes bubonic plague (1894).

B. Definitions

A-groove (P-groove, E-groove) These are sites on the surface of the ribosome (the protein-synthesizing complex in the cell) that bind the two RNA (ribonucleic acid) molecules (mRNA and tRNA) involved in the process of protein synthesis. "A" stands for "acceptor" site, "P" stands for "peptydyl" site, and "E" stands for "exit" site (see chapter II, section E, for further details).

A-B toxins One of two general types of toxins (poisons) produced by pathogens. This one is called an exotoxin and is composed of a subunit responsible for the poisonous effect (A) and a subunit responsible for binding to the host cell (B) it attacks.

ABO blood antigens All red blood cells have certain antigens on their surface that mark them as unique and that separate individuals into groups: A, B, AB, or O. The antigens are made up of glycolipids (sugars attached to lipids) and are important in some aspects of pathogenicity for unknown reasons (such as ulcers caused by *Helicobacter pylori* being found primarily in type O individuals).

Actinomycete A group of microorganisms that have characteristics both of bacteria and fungi, although many microbiologists characterize them as bacteria. Some produce long filaments and spores, while others are single celled. A subgroup of actinomycetes, known as streptomyces, produce most of the useful antibiotics for many infectious diseases, while two specific single-celled species are responsible for two dreaded diseases, tuberculosis and leprosy.

Adaptation In microorganisms, it is the ability to change the response of an entire population due to a change in environmental conditions, such as the presence of high concentrations of sugars, or low levels of oxygen. Both conditions temporarily delay growth but are eventually overcome. When the specific condition is removed, the entire population changes back to its original state. This is not a genetic change but is nevertheless important in how pathogens can "adapt" to some shifting environmental conditions.

Adenocarcinoma A malignant tumor originating in the epithelial (surface) tissue of glands. It is the most common type of colorectal cancer in the world and can be initiated by long-term infection with *Helicobacter pylori*, the microorganism that causes ulcers (see chapter V, section E, for further details).

Adhesin A structural part of the microorganism that is used to bind various surfaces. In pathogenic systems, these structures enable the organism to stick to specific cells, ultimately injecting their toxins or being "swallowed" into the cell itself. An important initial aspect of virulence.

Aflatoxin A strong toxin produced by a number of species of a specific fungus called *Aspergillus*. They can contaminate peanuts and other grains.

AIDS Acquired immunodeficiency syndrome, the wasting disease caused by the human immunodeficiency virus.

Alveoli Very small air sacs within the lungs, where the exchange of oxygen and carbon dioxide occurs. There are approximately 300 million alveoli in the lungs. Important in lung infections by various pathogens.

Amino acid Building blocks or subunits of proteins. There are twenty common amino acids that make up most proteins.

Anabolism A metabolic process that uses the chemical energy obtained by the breakdown of various foods such as sugars and fats to build (or synthesize) the structures of all cells, including bacteria.

Anthrax An infectious disease of animals, transmittable to man and caused by the microorganism *Bacillus anthracis*. It caused the only bioterror attack that ever occurred in the United States (soon after 9/11). (See chapter VII).

Antibiotic A chemical substance produced by one microorganism, capable of destroying or inhibiting the growth of another microorganism in very low concentration.

Antibody A class of proteins known as immunoglobulins, produced by our immune system (see B lymphocytes, also plasma cells) in response to a specific invasive substance (known as an antigen) that reacts specifically with that substance.

Anticodon A sequence of three nucleotides (building blocks of nucleic acids) in a small RNA molecule known as tRNA that complements a particular codon in a longer RNA known as mRNA (see chapter II, section E, for further details).

Antigen Any chemical substance that stimulates the production of antibodies by the immune system and reacts with a specific antibody.

Antigenic drift Usually small changes that occur in the chemical structure of surface antigens of a virus (such as influenza) that necessitate new antibodies to be generated in order to react with them. Earlier antibodies are therefore only partially protective or even unreactive (see chapter V, section F).

Antigenic shift An abrupt, major change in the chemical structure of surface antigens of a virus, due to mutation and selection that produces a different antigen, also necessitating the generation of new antibodies (see chapter V, section F).

Aspergillus A type of fungus that can produce a strong toxin (known as aflatoxin) that grows on various grains.

Asymptomatic An infection that causes no outward or observable symptoms, at least not initially.

AT base pairs "A" stands for adenine (a purine); "T" stands for thymine (a pyrimidine). Two of the chemical bases that join together naturally by hydrogen bonding in the DNA double helix.

Auxotroph(y) A nutritional mutant that requires a particular metabolite (amino acid, vitamin, etc.) that its parent strain from which it was derived (called a "wild type") does not.

AZT drug One of the first successful drugs that was used to treat AIDS patients. Its chemical name is Azidothymidine.

B lymphocyte A lymphocyte that has been induced to differentiate into a cell that can secrete antibodies.

BabA The most common adhesin (gluelike) protein that enables *Helicobacter pylori* (which causes ulcers) to adhere to intestinal epithelial cells. "O"-type individuals are most susceptible to this binding.

Bacillus anthracis The organism that causes anthrax, of which there are three kinds: cutaneous (skin), inhalation, and gastrointestinal anthrax.

Bacteriophage (phages) A virus that infects bacteria (often shortened to "phages").

BCG vaccine A vaccine used primarily in Europe but not in the United States. Named after the two Belgian scientists, Calmette and Guerin, who developed it (Bacille Calmette Guerin). It is derived from a strain of tuberculosis that infects cattle (*Mycobacterium bovis*) but not humans to any great extent, yet it produces strong immunity to the human tuberculosis organism (*Mycobacterium tuberculosis*).

Beta hemolysis A clear zone of red blood cell lysis around a bacterial colony growing on a blood-ager plate (petri dish). Usually associated with streptococcal infections.

Biofilm A "community" of microorganisms (of one or many species), surrounded by a thick gluey polysaccharide (sugar) shield.

Bioinformatics A relatively new technology that analyzes (by computers) the base sequences of genes to ascertain when they may function or not.

Bioterrorism The use of biological sources of all kinds (intact organisms or their products) as a weapon to kill, maim, and otherwise terrorize human populations, or to destroy plants and livestock.

Botulism A deadly disease caused by a potent toxin produced by the organism *Clostridium botulinum*, which produces paralysis in those who inadvertently swallow it, usually by consuming spoiled canned food.

Broad host range The ability of a "plasmid" (an extrachromosomal circular DNA factor found probably in all microorganisms—not a virus, though) that can be transmitted to many other species of microorganisms by conjugation or infection.

Broad spectrum Refers to the ability of an antibiotic to inhibit the growth of or kill a wide range of microorganisms.

Bubonic plague A devastating disease caused by the organism *Yersinia pestis*, which is transmitted from infected animals (usually rodents) by the bite of an infected flea. In medieval times, it wiped out a quarter of the population of Europe.

CagA toxin One of the principal toxins produced by the ulcer-causing pathogen *Helicobacter pylori*, which may expedite the penetration of another toxin (VacA) into host epithelial cells. Not all strains of *Helicobacter* produce both toxins.

Capsule An extracellular coat surrounding many microorganisms, usually polysaccharide in nature, that can act to protect certain pathogens, such as *Streptococcus pneumoniae*, from being destroyed by phagocytosis.

Carbuncle A type of deep-seeded infection usually caused by staphylococci that invades the skin and tissue underneath the skin (subcutaneous), producing a cluster of painful boils.

Catabolism A subtype of metabolism in which chemical energy is produced by the stepwise chemical breakdown of certain foodstuffs such as sugars and fats. Part of the energy that is produced can be stored and used to synthesize important structural components of the cell in "anabolic" reactions.

Catalase An enzyme produced by many but not all microorganisms, which can destroy hydrogen peroxide, a poisonous end product of metabolism that would be fatal to the cell unless it were destroyed.

Catheter A thin, flexible tube inserted into some bodily duct or cavity to enable external fluids to be infused there. They also permit drainage of the bodily cavity or duct. Prone to infection by opportunistic bacteria.

CD4 lymphocyte A type of white blood cell that is involved in controlling the sequence of events leading to the production of antibodies and other active cells that interact with or inactivate infectious antigens such as pathogens. They display receptor sites (CD4 markers) on their surface to initiate the process. However, these receptors also bind the HIV virus (which causes AIDS), which is why the immune system becomes defective as the CD4 lymphocytes are gradually destroyed or inactivated.

CDC (Centers for Disease Control and Treatment) This is the primary governmental oversight organization that operates various departments to monitor occupational safety and various health issues, such as publicizing disease outbreaks, treatment protocols and references (such as availability of vaccines), etc. Their laboratory complex is in Atlanta, Georgia.

Cholera An infection of the small intestine by the organism *Vibrio cholerae*, whose toxins cause a large amount of liquid diarrhea; can be fatal because of extreme dehydration.

Ciproflaxin antibiotic A relatively new antibiotic that became "famous" by being used in the anthrax bioterror attack of 2001. However, it can be used to treat many bacterial infections.

Clostridium botulinum The microorganism that causes botulism, by producing an extremely potent toxin. Usually found in spoiled canned vegetables that have not been heated in a vacuum long enough to destroy the spores that it produces.

Clostridium tetani The microorganism that produces tetanus (or lockjaw), a disease that is usually initiated by deep wounds or punctures, where the organism can thrive and produce a potent toxin that destroys the nervous system. Its most common symptoms are spasms in the jaw muscles, which results in its tightening. Its common name is "lockjaw."

Coagulase An enzyme produced by a variety of microorganisms, including pathogens, and in particular *Staphylococcus aureus*, that converts the soluble form of the clotting factor called fibrinogen to fibrin, which then coats the pathogen, making it difficult for phagocytosis by white blood cells. A specific assay for coagulase has been developed to determine whether it is produced in a staphylococcal infection. If so, the infection is characterized as "coagulase positive" and dangerous.

Codon A sequence of three nucleotides in a messenger RNA (mRNA) that complements another sequence of three nucleotides in a transfer RNA (tRNA) (anticodon), according to the base pairing rules of the Watson-Crick double helix (A-T, G-C). Each codon specifies a particular amino acid in the process of protein synthesis.

Collagenase An enzyme produced by many microorganisms, including some pathogens, that degrades or breaks down the largest single protein component of the body—namely, collagen, which is the primary component of bones. It therefore can be characterized as a virulence factor produced by a number of pathogens to aid in their penetration of the host to exert their toxic effects.

Colony In microbiological terms, a colony is a large number of cells, all descendent from one cell, that were deposited on a hardened nutrient agar plate (petri dish). It is visible to the naked eye, it can contain millions of individual bacterial cells, and its shape (round, irregular) and consistency (mucoid, rough, smooth) are valuable as diagnostic tools.

Complete medium A nutrient growth solution that contains all the necessary energy sources and growth factor for cultivation of most microorganisms, including nutritional (auxotrophic) mutants that are unable to synthesize one or more metabolites that are supplied by the "complete" medium.

Confocal microscope A relatively new type of microscope that uses a laser beam to visualize specific planes in a thick specimen. After visualization, computer analysis can assemble a three-dimensional image of the structure. Has been of particular use in the visualization of biofilms (cities of microbes—see chapter VI).

Conjugation A type of gene transfer in microorganisms that requires contact between cells and in which a large number of genes can be transferred from one conjugant (male) to another (female).

Constitutive enzyme An enzyme that is always synthesized in a cell. Usually refers to "housekeeping" enzymes that are required to maintain the cell constantly (e.g., enzymes involved in nucleic acid synthesis).

Cord factor A unique component of the cell wall of *Mycobacterium tuberculosis*, which causes human TB. It is one of the virulence factors of the pathogen known as a surface "glycolypid," influencing the organism to grow in "serpentine" cords in the test tube. It is toxic when extracted and injected by itself into mice.

Corepressor A small molecule that binds to a repressor that is inactive and activates it so that the latter can bind to a region of an operon (called the operator), which then prevents the enzyme that synthesizes mRNA (RNA polymerase) from binding to start transcription of the structural genes of the operon (see chapter II, section F).

Corona virus A virus group containing a new corona virus that in 2003 was identified as the cause of SARS (severe acute respiratory syndrome). Initially isolated in China and spread to many countries, it was feared that a pandemic would ensue, but by quick action of the international community, the disease was contained and virtually disappeared within a year.

Corynebacterium diphtheriae The causative agent of diphtheria, a highly contagious disease characterized by a severe constriction of the air passages due to the production of the diphtheria toxin. Vaccination is the prime preventative method, but through lapses, it flares up in developed and Third World countries.

Cryptic mutation A mutation in which no outward signs of change are evident.

Cryptococcus neoformans A devastating disease of the brain, caused by a yeast, and one of the four most prevalent diseases found in AIDS patients whose immune system has broken down. It is almost 100% fatal when expressed. The infection occurs in the meninges, or the lining of the brain.

Cutaneous anthrax The most common of the three types of anthrax infections, in which a large necrotic (degradation) region occurs on the skin, usually the arms, after spores on an animal's body (usually a sheep) are deposited in a cut or small abrasion, followed by germination. Most cases are cured by antibiotic treatment.

Cytokine Small protein molecules produced by certain cells of the immune system (such as lymphocytes) that can affect the behavior of other cells of the immune system (such as macrophages) by binding to them (cytokine receptors). This binding then enhances the ability of the macrophages to ingest invading pathogens, as well as attracting other types of white blood cells to increase the inflammatory response.

Delayed hypersensitivity A type of allergic response common in some chronic diseases, such as tuberculosis, in which cytokine-stimulated cells of the immune system damage other cells and tissues of the body because they are constantly being stimulated to try to destroy the pathogen but instead produce an excess of inflammatory factors, which act detrimentally.

DNA (deoxyribonucleic acid) The macromolecule in the cell that stores genetic information in its sequence of building blocks, purines, and pyrimidines.

DNA polymerase The primary enzyme that all cells use to synthesize DNA. There are a number of different DNA polymerases, which have different functions during the synthetic process.

Double helix The structural form of DNA, consisting of one helix wound around the other. However, in nature there are other such helices besides DNA.

E-groove (see A-groove).

Ebola virus A deadly virus (of which there are four types) named after a river in Africa where it was first identified, which causes a hemorrhagic disease of humans and primates in which the entire circulatory system hemorrhages, leaking blood out into the body. It is highly contagious, fatal, and spread by infected blood.

Endocarditis An inflammation of the heart valves or lining of the heart, caused in many cases by infection with a number of different types of bacterial pathogens, such as streptococci, although fungi can sometimes also be the cause.

Endocytosis An engulfment process by which cells take up bacteria, viruses, or any other "insoluble" particle by encircling them in a vesicle that is derived from the cell membrane itself.

Endotoxin A structural component of a number of pathogens that is part of the cell surface, known as LPS (or lipopolysaccharide). It is toxic for those who are infected, causing high fever, shock, inflammation, and low blood pressure.

Enzyme A biological catalyst that controls the rate and extent of chemical (metabolic) reactions in the cell. All enzymes are proteins, but many are controlled by small nonprotein cofactors or minerals that expedite their function in converting the "substrate" into the final end product.

Erysipelas A skin infection (usually the face and lower limbs) caused primarily by a streptococcal organism (*Streptococcus pyogenes*). The symptoms include blisters; swollen, red, and warm skin; fever; and chills. Often occurs in infants and young children.

Escherichia coli A common, mostly harmless, inhabitant of the intestine, often associated with fecal contamination if found in drinking water. However, they can cause bladder infections, and a new strain (O157) has been implicated in a severe gastroenteritis.

Eukaryotic cell Refers to the complex cell type found in all multicellular organisms, consisting of a nucleus and other organelles involved in maintaining its existence.

Exotoxin A soluble toxin secreted from many pathogens, usually proteinaceous in nature, that exerts deadly effects on host cells.

Feedback inhibition A control mechanism existing in all cells, in which the end product of a particular metabolic pathway can shut the pathway down by inhibiting the activity (not the synthesis) of the first enzyme in the pathway. Also called end product inhibition.

Feedback loop Refers to the "circular" model described above for feedback inhibition.

Fermentation The catabolic metabolic process in a particular microorganism, where energy sources from food, mostly carbohydrates (sugars), are chemically broken down anaerobically (without oxygen) in a stepwise manner to produce an end product that is an economically useful organic compound, such as alcohol. Fermentation is the basis for industrial microbiology.

Fibrin The insoluble protein involved in the clotting of blood. Some pathogens can convert the precursor of fibrin—fibrinogen—to fibrin, which then coats its surface, inhibiting phagocytosis.

Fimbra (fimbrae, pl.) A type of appendage sticking out of cells that enables them to stick to a specific surface.

Flagellum (flagella, pl.) The organelle of locomotion in prokaryotic cells, consisting of one contractile protein called flagellin, that allows the microorganism to move. Flagella exist within the eukaryotic cell kingdom as well.

Fungus (fungi, pl.) A large group of microorganisms that grow mostly as strands in their microenvironment, produce spores, and are eukaryotic in the sense that their strands are "septate" (made up of cross walls and individual cells), containing a nucleus. They are divided into four groups depending on the type of spore sac they produce. Pathogenic fungi exist and are extremely difficult to treat, especially if their infection is internal (within the body). Yeasts are fungi that have lost their ability for strand-like growth.

Furuncle A skin infection (also called a boil), usually caused by *Staphylococcus aureus*, that starts by infection of hair follicles anywhere on the body. Without treatment the infection becomes deeper into the skin and subcutaneous tissues and leads to a carbuncle.

Gastric acid The acid secreted in the stomach (mostly HCl) that helps digest food.

Gastrointestinal tract Includes the entire digestive system, starting with the mouth and proceeding to the esophagus, the stomach, and the small and large intestines.

GC base pair "G" stands for guanine (a purine), and "C" stands for cytosine (a pyrimidine). Two of the chemical bases that join together naturally by hydrogen bonding in the DNA double helix.

Gene The fundamental unit of heredity, composed of a specific sequence of purine and pyrimidine bases that codes for a specific protein.

Genetic code A universal (all organisms, including pathogens, have essentially the same code) library by which genetic information encoded in DNA or RNA (by their sequence of bases) specifies the amino acid sequences of every protein.

Genotype The sum total of all the genes that constitute an individual multicellular or unicellular organism.

Genus A collection of related organisms, composed of a number of species. In practice, it is the first term in the binomial sequence of naming a specific organism (genus-species: e.g., *Streptococcus* [genus] *pyogenes* [species]).

Granuloma An expression of a chronic or long-term response to inflammation, consisting of a variety of different white blood cells, such as lymphocytes and macrophages. In TB, the granuloma is part of a tubercle that walls off live TB microorganisms like a "prison" to prevent them from spreading. They can last many years.

Group A streptococcus A form of *Streptococcus pyogenes* that secretes powerful toxins that lyse red blood cells and other cells. It is responsible for most cases of illness caused by streptococcus.

Guillain-Barre syndrome A rare disorder (1–2 out of 100,000 people) in which a person's own immune system can damage peripleral nerve cells and cause muscle weakness. It is manifested after an acute infection such as flu but is rarely fatal.

Helicobacter The genus that includes the organism causing ulcers, *Helicobacter pylori.*

Helicobacter pylori See *Helicobacter* above.

Hemagglutinin In general terms, hemagglutinin is a glycoprotein that agglutinates (clumps) red blood cells. In specific terms, it is one of two types of "spikes" that project out from the surface of flu viruses, essential for attaching to specific host cell receptors. The hemagglutinin (HA) spike also agglutinates red blood cells, which is why it is called "hemagglutinin." This property has been useful in delineating different "subtypes" of different flu viruses.

Hemoglobin The primary protein complex of red blood cells, whose function is to carry oxygen.

Hemolysin In general pathogenic terms, it is a type of toxin (there are a number of subtypes) that lyses or destroys red blood cells. Hemolysins are detected by the type of zone of clearing around a colony growing on a nutrient agar plate infused with red blood cells.

Hemophilus influenzae An opportunistic pathogen that can cause a number of different types of pneumonia and meningitis. It was mistakenly thought also to cause influenza in early studies (up until 1933) because it appeared as a secondary invader after the onset of the flu (hence its species name—*influenzae*).

Heterozygous A "genetic" condition where two different forms of the same gene can exist on homologous chromosomes. One could be "dominant" over the other (called recessive).

Host-parasite relationship The "modern" definition of a pathogen, in which the invading microorganism can exist in several relationships: (1) causing the disease, (2) being destroyed by the host, or (3) existing in the host without being destroyed.

Housekeeping gene A simile for "constitutive," a gene that is always being expressed because it is essential for life (such as genes involved in DNA synthesis).

Hyaluronidase An enzyme produced as a "toxin" by a number of pathogens, such as staphylococci and streptococci, that degrades hyaluronic acid, an important constituent of connective tissue. As such it aids the pathogens in penetrating inner bodily sites. Amazingly enough, it can also be used therapeutically to help other drugs penetrate the skin for uptake by the body.

Hydrogen bonding A weak chemical attraction between a positively charged hydrogen atom of one compound and a negatively charged atom of another compound. Of extreme importance in "holding" together the double helix of DNA, by maintaining the bonding between the two types of base pairs: AT (which has two hydrogen bonds) and GC (which has three hydrogen bonds).

Immunoglobulin A class of glyco (sugar) proteins that comprise the five distinct types of antibodies: IgG, IgA, IgM, IgD, and IgE. All except IgE are involved in interacting with pathogens as well as numerous other antigens. IgE is involved with those antigens that cause allergies.

Impetigo A contagious skin infection that produces blisters and sores, caused by a number of pathogens but in particular *Staphylococcus aureus* or *Streptococcus pyogenes*—common in infants.

Inhalation anthrax A severe form of anthrax in which spores are deposited through the nasal passage to the lungs, where they germinate, are phagocytized by macrophages (but are not killed), are transported to lymph nodes, and invade the blood stream. Powerful toxins are secreted by the pathogen *Bacillus anthracis*, which can kill the victim within forty-eight hours. Fortunately, such anthrax is rare, although in the bioterror attack eleven out of a possible thirty thousand exposures developed this lethal type.

In vitro Any study that is performed under conditions not involving a living organism; namely, in a test tube or other receptacle.

In vivo Any study that is performed in a living organism rather than in a test tube or other receptacle.

Inducible enzyme Any enzyme that is synthesized under the control of a small, nonproteinaceous molecule, provided that the substrate (the substance on which the enzyme reacts) is present.

Induction (in enzyme synthesis) The genetic and metabolic process by which an inducible enzyme is synthesized.

Inflammation An immune response to infection or injury, characterized by heat, swelling, redness, and soreness at the affected site.

Influenza (flu) An acute infectious disease of the respiratory tract, caused by a virus, of which there are three main types: A, B, and C, of which type A is the most severe in humans.

Initiation (in protein synthesis) The beginning of the metabolic process by which genes are expressed, starting with the synthesis of messenger (m) RNA.

Integrase enzyme (in viruses) The general name for a class of enzymes that control the "integration" of viral DNA into the host chromosome (both in eukaryotic and prokaryotic cells).

Integration (in viruses) The insertion of viral genes into a host genome under the control of the integrase and other enzymes. In prokaryotes, the process is called lysogeny. In eukaryotics, the process is called latent.

Invasins A particular class of adhesin molecules that promote penetration by the pathogen into host cells and tissues. They bind to host cell receptors to initiate the process.

Kaposi sarcoma Usually a rare tumor that erupts on the skin, but which began to appear in large numbers in young men with AIDS. It was so common that it became a condition that defined who had AIDS, and it was responsible for stimulating research that led to the discovery of the HIV virus that causes AIDS.

Koch's postulates A set of four rules used to determine the specific cause of an infectious disease, first proposed by R. Koch in the nineteenth century and still relevant today for determining whether a specific microorganism causes a specific disease.

Lassa fever virus One of the deadly hemorrhagic fever viruses, commonly concentrated in the tropics (first detected in 1969). Characterized by massive leakage of fluid from the circulatory system, causing shock, neurological defects, and, eventually, death. It is spread by a species of rat found only in West Africa, through airborne droplets from rat urine or contaminated food.

Latent infection In eukaryotic viral infections, the viral state in which the virus is "hidden" by its integration into a site on the host chromosome. It produces no new virus particles, but at any time it can be "activated" and return to a "growth" cycle whereby new viruses are produced.

Lecithinase An enzyme that can degrade lecithin (a fatty substance composed of a number of components, including fatty acids, choline, phosphoric acid, phospholipids, and other components). It is part of the cell membrane and is involved in protecting cells from harmful oxidation, as well as being part of the protective covering surrounding the brain. A number of pathogens degrade lecithin as part of their invasive process to penetrate regions of the body.

Leprosy An ancient disease caused by the organism *Mycobacterium leprae*. Characterized by eventual extensive lesions all over the body if left untreated. It is still endemic in Southeast Asia and India.

Leukocidin A bacterial toxin that can destroy white blood cells. *Staphylococcus aureus* is a potent producer of the toxin, which consists of two proteins.

Light microscope A microscope that employs visible light to resolve and observe microscopic objects.

Lymphocyte A type of white blood cell with a large nucleus, which has many functions involved in active immunity (the generation of an immune response through the production of antibodies or other cytotoxic lymphocytes).

Lymph nodes Various sites in the body that consist of a small "organelle"-like structure where all the "players" of the immune system and the infectious antigens (pathogens) are concentrated together to enable them to interact. It is also the site where the blood circulatory system connects to the lymph circulatory system.

Lymphoma A cancer that arises in the lymphatic system. In *Helicobacter* infections it can be a consequence of long-term (or chronic) infections due to the expression of inflammatory factors in about 20% of the cases.

Lysogenic conversion An alteration in the property or properties of a microorganism that has integrated a bacterial virus (called a prophage) into its chromosome.

Lysogeny The condition in which a microorganism integrates a bacterial virus (prophage) into its chromosome.

Lytic infection A typical result of bacterial virus (phage) infection of a sensitive bacterial cell, where the injected genetic material of the virus (DNA or RNA) takes over the control of the host cell to produce new parts of the virus, which are then packaged together (maturation) to produce the full, intact virus. The intact virus then lyses (destroys the cell from within). Usually from one infecting bacterial virus, approximately two hundred new viruses can be produced and liberated from the lysed cell.

Macromolecule A large molecule composed of repeating subunits. Four of the most common macromolecules are nucleic acids (DNA and RNA), proteins (amino acids), carbohydrates (sugars), and lipids (fatty acids).

Mad cow disease An infectious neurological disease of cattle, caused by abnormal proteins called "prions" that accumulate in the brain, eventually causing spongelike "holes" or gaps in the network of neurons (nerve cells). Humans can catch this disease, which takes many years to develop, by eating infected beef.

Marburg virus A hemorrhagic disease virus very similar to Ebola, endemic to regions of Africa, that affects humans and primates. It was named after the German town in which it was first found (Marburg), which occurred when technicians handled "infected" primates imported from Africa. Symptoms include fever, chills, fatigue, rash, and, finally, hemorrhaging from the circulatory system.

Meningitis In general terms, this is a disease in which the lining of the brain, the meninges, is affected. The main pathogenic cause is *Neisseria meningitidis*, although *Streptococcus pneumoniae* (which causes pneumonia) and *Hemophilus influenzae* can also cause the disease.

Messenger RNA (mRNA) A single-stranded, long RNA macromolecule synthesized under control of a DNA template, which is the beginning of transcription during the process of protein synthesis.

Metabolism The sum total of all the metabolic processes (chemical pathways) in the cell, encompassing anabolism and catabolism.

Microbiome A diverse group of more than 100 trillion microbes that cooperate with the cells of the body to keep humans healthy.

Minimal medium A sparse nutrient-growth medium that contains an organic energy source (such as sugar), a nitrogen source in the form of a salt (ammonium sulphate), and other minerals. This medium cannot support the growth of biochemical mutants (auxotrophs) that require an organic growth factor (such as an amino acid or vitamin) for such proliferation, but it can support the growth of its parent (wild type) strain from which it was derived.

Monocistronic message An mRNA molecular that codes for one gene.

M-protein Proteins found in the cell surface of pathogenic streptococci that are involved in its pathogenicity.

Multiple myeloma A cancer of the stem or plasma cells of the bone marrow.

Mutation A spontaneous and undirected change in the sequence of bases in a gene that leads to a new genotype by altering the protein that is encoded by the gene.

Mycobacterium avium Causes bird TB.

Mycobacterium bovis Causes animal TB.

Mycobacterium leprae Causes leprosy.

Mycobacterium marinus Causes TB-like disease in fishes.

Mycobacterium tuberculosis Causes human TB.

Narrow spectrum Describes an antibiotic that can inhibit only a small number of pathogens.

Natural selection The selection by the environment of the "fittest" organism for that environment.

Nef (rev, tat, vif, vpr) Transcription factors produced by "splicing" in the further maturation (developmental) process of the HIV virus that causes AIDS (see chapter V, section B).

Neuraminidase An enzyme that cleaves sugars that are linked to an organic acid (neuraminic acid). In pathogenic terms, the most common are the viral neuraminidases of the influenza (flu) virus, which make up one of two "spikes" on the surface of the virus that aids the virus in attaching to its host cell. The neuraminidase degrades the mucous of the respiratory tract. The neuraminidase (NA for short) can mutate easily and is responsible along with the other spike (hemagglutinin) for producing new flu viruses from season to season. At least nine types of influenza neuraminidase have been identified.

Nucleocapsid A protein container composed of many subunits that encase the tightly packed nucleic acid within the virus itself.

Nucleotide An organic molecule that constitutes the backbone of nucleic acids composed of a purine or pyrimidine base, linked to a sugar (ribose or deoxyribose) and a phosphate group.

Operator A nucleotide region situated immediately to the right (downstream) of another nucleotide region called the promoter, to which the repressor protein can bind to prevent the attachment of RNA polymerase required for transcription. The two regions are part of the "operon" (see chapter II, section F).

Operon The functional regulatory control system in microorganisms, consisting of structural genes (those genes that express the synthesis of a particular enzyme in a metabolic pathway) and regulatory genes (those genes that control the functioning of the structural genes). All these genes are in regions that are adjacent to each other on the bacterial chromosome. Another regulatory gene situated at some distance from the organized region is responsible for expressing the protein repressor (see chapter II, section F).

Opportunistic pathogen A potential pathogen that can express its pathogenicity in hosts with defective immune systems or as a secondary invader after the primary pathogen has weakened the host in other ways.

Osteomyelitis A sudden or chronic inflammatory condition of the bone that erupts as a secondary consequence of bacterial infection, most notably with *Streptococcus pyogenes* that comes from the blood.

Overlapping genes The ability of one sequence of bases in a gene to code for more than one protein. Common in viruses where the entire small genome could be seriously compromised without this feature (see chapter V, section B, on AIDS).

Pandemic An epidemic that spreads worldwide due to infection by bacterial or viral pathogens.

Passive immunity Rapid immunity to an infectious pathogen, by transfer of serum containing resistance (antibodies) to that infection already present from animals or other individuals.

Pasteurization A heating process for foods (liquid or solid) for a short time at a temperature below boiling, so as to kill potential pathogens or lower their number without damaging the food.

Pathogen Microorganism (including viruses) capable of causing a specific disease in a host.

Pathogenicity island Segments of a chromosome in a pathogen that are grouped together, containing a number of virulence genes. Some pathogens contain more than one "island."

Penicillium notatum A "famous" fungus that produces penicillin, the first useful antibiotic ever discovered, for treating a number of bacterial infections, including those of streptococci and staphylococci.

Pepsin An enzyme released into the stomach acid that degrades foods into fragments of proteins (peptides).

Persistent infection In viral infections, the virus is reproduced in the cell over a long period of time without lysing (destroying) the cell from within, so that it can be released from the surface of the cell for this longer period, thus increasing the numbers of new viruses.

Persistor cells Certain bacterial cells present in a biofilm grow (multiply) very slowly and are therefore not as sensitive to treatment by antibiotics or other drugs that usually act on growing cells more efficiently. As a result, they survive and can reform the biofilm after the faster-growing sensitive cells are destroyed. Thus, the biofilm becomes more resistant to treatment because a greater percentage of the persistor cells are present.

P-groove (see A-groove).

Phagocytosis A prime function of the immune system, carried out by certain white blood cells (e.g., macrophages that ingest invading pathogens and destroy them within the "phagocyte").

Pharyngitis An inflammation of the pharynx or the throat (often called a sore throat), which is caused mostly by infection with pathogenic streptococci or viruses.

Phase variation A spontaneous and common alteration in the expression of surface attachment structures in microorganisms, due to the random switching on and switching off of genes that are included in producing them. This is an important mechanism by which certain pathogens can resist the immune reaction, by forcing the system that had been induced to inactivate one surface structure to be reinduced to react with a new, different one.

Phenotype The physical or observable expression of the genotype, which is not always expressed.

Pili Thin, hairlike structures on many bacteria that are involved in a number of functions, such as attachment to other cells or in genetic conjugation. An important property of pathogens to enable them to attach to their specific host cells.

Planktonic cell Free-living bacterial cells that are capable of forming a biofilm by attaching to a specific surface and becoming immobilized.

Plasma cell The end product of the differentiation of a B lymphocyte capable of synthesizing and secreting antibodies.

Pneumocystis carinii A severe, pneumonia-like lung disease caused by a minute fungus whose spores lodge in the lung. It was one of the leading causes of death of AIDS sufferers during the beginning of the AIDS epidemic.

Pneumonia A lung disease involving congestion of air sacs, which can be caused by a number of different primary and opportunistic pathogens. However, most of the cases are caused by *Streptococcus pneumoniae.*

Polio (infantile paralysis) A contagious viral disease caused by the polio virus on which nerves of the central nervous system (brain and spinal cord) are destroyed, leading to paralysis. Most individuals are resistant to polio after becoming infected (subclinical). Several vaccines developed in the late 1950s and 1960s have helped tremendously in reducing the number of cases worldwide.

Polycistronic message An mRNA that transcribes more than one gene.

Primary pathogen A pathogen (bacterial or viral) that is capable of causing a specific disease in a healthy individual with a healthy immune system.

Prime (3' to 5' or 5' to 3') (in DNA) A shorthand term to describe the direction of each strand of the double helix, one progressing 3' to 5'; the other, 5' to 3'. The numbers refer to specific carbon atoms in the sugar (deoxyribose) that forms part of the backbone of DNA.

Prokaryotic Refers to all bacteria that exist as single cells that do not possess a nucleus but are surrounded by a membrane and rigid cell wall. However they do possess a "nucleoid," which contains the genetic material (DNA) without a nuclear membrane.

Prophage The latent state of a bacterial virus whose entire genome (chromosome) is integrated into the much-larger bacteria chromosome and multiplies with it once each division cycle.

Proteomics The analysis of the complete protein makeup of the cell that is expressed by the genotype.

Pseudomonas aeruginosa An opportunistic pathogen that can be deadly in a variety of infections and genetically based syndromes, such as cystic fibrosis, an inherited disease that causes mucous to clog the lungs.

Purine One of the two types of molecules that compose part of the structure of nucleic acids. They are called adenine and guanine.

Pyrimidine One of three types of molecules that compose part of the structure of nucleic acids. They are thymine, uracil, and cytosine.

Quorum sensing A form of chemical "communication" between bacteria, mediated by small molecules that permit them to determine their total number or to activate certain genes when this number is reached. The phenomenon has been studied extensively during the formation of biofilms.

Receptor site In general microbiological germs, these are sites on the surface of bacteria or viruses that allow specific parts of the site (usually a membrane protein) to bind to molecules in the milieu surrounding the microorganism, so that they can adapt to environmental conditions.

Recombination (crossing over) A process by which new combinations of genes are created on a chromosome due to the phenomenon of "crossing over" between a set of homologous (or similar) chromosomes or their parts. One of the two hallmarks of evolution, together with mutation and selection.

Regulatory gene A gene that controls the functioning of other genes, either by controlling its rate of expression or whether or not it is expressed at all.

Replisome The complex of enzymes and control factors in all organisms that are involved in activating DNA replication at the initiation site of such replication. It also controls the movement of the replication fork that travels around the DNA until the entire macromolecule is replicated.

Repression The term applied to the regulation of specific metabolic pathways by certain proteins that inactivate the synthesis of such pathways.

Repressor The protein molecule that is involved in repression. It has a different chemical structure for different repressible systems.

Reverse transcriptase A remarkable enzyme, first discussed in the 1970s, that synthesizes double-stranded DNA complementary to a RNA template. Most prevalent in viruses that have RNA as their genetic material (e.g., HIV).

Reye's syndrome A mostly fatal syndrome that affects the brain and liver, which occurs primarily in children who are given aspirin for treatment of pain and fever in influenza or chicken pox infections.

Rhinovirus The main cause of the common cold, of which there are many types.

Ribosomal RNA (rRNA) Several types of RNA that are structurally part of the ribosome involved in protein synthesis.

Ribosome The protein-synthesizing factory of every cell (prokaryotic and eukaryotic). Thousands of ribosomes are present in cells to carry out this process. It is composed of RNA and many types of proteins.

Ribozyme RNA molecules that can act as enzymes.

Rickettsia A small bacterium that has lost some of its metabolic "strength" so that it can survive only within a living cell (like viruses). They are the cause of a number of deadly diseases, including typhus and Rocky Mountain spotted fever, and are transmitted by mites or ticks.

Rickettsia prowazekii The cause of epidemic typhus.

Rickettsia rickettsii The cause of Rocky Mountain spotted fever, spread by the bite of insects usually ticks.

RNA (abbreviation for ribonucleic acid) One of two types of nucleic acids.

RNA polymerase The enzyme that synthesizes RNA under direction of a template, which can either be DNA or RNA itself. There are a number of different types of RNA polymerase.

SabA A type of surface adhesin that is produced by *Helicobacter pylori* (the organism that causes ulcers) in a transient "gene-switching" process from the normal adhesin, BabA, to thwart phagocytosis.

Salmonella typhimurium A type of typhoid (an acute infection of a number of organs) that occurs in mice and other rodents. Since the mouse pathogen doesn't infect humans, it has become a useful model to study a number of genetic and molecular aspects of typhoid itself.

SARS (severe acute respiratory syndrome) A viral respiratory disease caused by a new "corona virus" that first appeared in 2003 in China and spread quickly to thirty-seven countries. Symptoms include high fever, body aches, and lung congestion resembling pneumonia. It is highly contagious and is spread by a variety of ways, including personal contact, sneezing, and touching surfaces that are contaminated.

Scalded skin syndrome A severe skin infection, primarily in babies and young children, in which the skin actually is flaked off, caused primarily by pathogenic staphylococci. The effect is due to an exotoxin produced by the pathogen.

Scarlet fever A disease caused by an exotoxin released from group A streptococci, usually after the onset of a sore throat or pharyngitis if it is not treated. A rash that first appears on the neck and chest and then spreads is the most common feature of the disease.

Scrapie virus A fatal neurodegenerative disease of sheep and goats, caused by a prion, the abnormal protein that produces spongelike holes in the brain. It probably was transmitted in infected feed eaten by cows, producing the first cases of mad cow disease in the 1970s and 1980s.

Secretion In microorganisms, the metabolic process that controls the elimination of products from the cytoplasm through the cell membrane and cell wall. Many proteins are involved in the process, which is sequential in nature.

Semiconservative (replication) A characterization of the DNA replication process that occurs in most organisms, in which each original strand of the double helix is preserved as the template while new strands are "polymerized" against each template (one old strand, one new strand).

Serotype A specific strain of a microorganism that has surface antigens that are different from those on other strains.

Serum A liquid fraction of the blood that is present after the removal of the red blood cells and other clotting substances. It is the main source of antibodies and the soluble factors that are involved in the immune reaction.

Siderophore A complex found in many bacteria that sequesters (removes or binds) iron after infection. It competes better with host complexes (ferritin) that also complex iron.

Species The ultimate definition of an organism, which consists of a group of individuals that can breed actually or potentially with each other but are isolated from any other group in this respect. In microorganisms, it is the second name given to describe a specific organism, the first being the genus.

Splicing A molecular process whereby certain newly synthesized mRNA products in a microorganism are "cut" further by special enzymes to provide new mRNAs for coding smaller additional proteins. A very important example of this process occurs in the HIV virus that causes AIDS.

Staphylococcus A large group of sphere-like microorganisms that resemble "grape-like" clusters under the light microscope, some of whose members cause a large number of external diseases (usually on the skin) by producing a large variety of exotoxins.

Staphylococcus aureus The "archetype" pathogen of the staphylococci responsible for most of the diseases it causes.

Streptococcus A large group of sphere-like microorganisms that exist mostly as short or long snakelike chains (to differentiate them crudely from the staphylococci) under the light microscope, most of whose members cause a large number of internal diseases by producing a large variety of exotoxins.

Streptococcus mutans Involved in causing tooth decay.

Streptococcus pyogenes The "archetype" pathogen of streptococci responsible for most of the diseases it causes.

Streptococcus pneumoniae An exception to the general chain-like pattern of streptococcil growth, existing mostly as "diplococci" (in twos) surrounded by an extensive polysaccharide (sugar) capsule. This pathogen causes over 85% of all cases of pneumonia.

Streptococcus viridans Causes endocarditis, a severe heart infection.

Streptolysins O and S Deadly exotoxins produced by pathogenic streptococci, which destroy not only red blood cells, but white blood cells, liver cells, and heart muscle cells as well.

Streptomycin The first useful antibiotic discovered that could inhibit the growth of *Mycobacterium tuberculosis*, the microorganism that causes TB.

Structural gene (in operon) Genes that code for specific enzymes in a metabolic pathway.

Substrate Any substance that interacts with a specific enzyme in the first step to modify or change it into a final end product.

Susceptibility (host) Describes the state of well-being of an individual (good, fair, poor), which will determine how successful an invading pathogen (including viruses) will be in causing a specific disease. There is a strong correlation between this "state" and that of the immune system (temporary or permanent). The more effective the immune system, the greater probability of a feeling of well-being.

Superantigens Powerful exotoxins produced by a number of pathogens that induce the immune system to act abnormally, resulting in the massive release of cytokines (inflammation-inducing factors) from certain lymphocytes called T-helper cells that cause toxic effects on tissues.

Superoxide dismutase An enzyme that is involved in repairing cells by degrading of "superoxides" to hydrogen peroxide, which is then destroyed by another enzyme catalase. Superoxides are damaging to the body (and bacteria), by forming what are called "free radicals."

Suppression A mutation in one gene that suppresses the expression of another mutation at another genic site to restore the original trait.

Tetanus A dangerous disease caused by *Clostridium tetani*. The organism produces a nerve-destroying toxin that paralyzes muscle fibers, usually beginning in the jaw.

T-helper cell A type of white blood cell (lymphocyte) involved in controlling the expression of antibodies after interacting with an antigen. It is also the primary cell infected by the HIV virus.

Toxic shock syndrome (TSS) A deadly disease in which toxins produced either by staphylococci or streptococci induce high fever, shock, and damage to a number of organs in the body.

Toxin Any poisonous substance produced by pathogens.

Transduction (generalized and specialized) One type of gene transfer between microorganisms that is mediated by a bacterial virus. The virus carries chromosome fragments from its destroyed host in its head structure and, after infecting a new host, integrates those fragments into the chromosome of the new host. Only a few genes can be "transduced" (see chapter II, section G).

Transcription The transfer of genetic information from being encoded in the DNA of a gene to a messenger RNA (mRNA) by the enzyme RNA polymerase.

Transfer RNA (tRNA) Small RNA molecules that combine with specific amino acids. Each tRNA binds to one amino acid.

Transformation (in bacteria) One type of gene transfer between microorganisms, in which DNA from one type (the donor) is incorporated (taken up) into another related cell type (the recipient) and becomes integrated into the chromosome of the recipient. Only a few genes are transformed.

Transformation (in viral cancer) An infection in which the virus does not lyse the host cell but instead becomes integrated into the host cell chromosome and somehow transforms that cell into a cancer cell. However, in other cases, long-term bacterial infections (such as chronic ulcers) can also induce transformation in human cells.

Translation The process by which genetic information in DNA is ultimately "translated" into a specific amino acid sequence of a protein on the ribosome.

Transposon Genes that can be moved from one DNA macromolecule to another in the same or other cells, under the control of specific enzymes called transposases.

Trypsin An enzyme in the stomach that degrades protein foodstuffs for digestion.

Tubercle A "castle"-like structure in the lung, called a granuloma, that surrounds live tuberculosis microorganisms to prevent them from spreading. Individuals can survive with tubercles for many years as long as the immune system is functioning.

Tuberculin test A hypersensitivity (allergy) test to determine whether an individual has been infected with the organism that causes tuberculosis. Injection of a very small amount of extract of the organism itself under the skin of infected individuals will result in a gradual reddening and a raised area within forty-eight to seventy-two hours.

Tuberculosis A devastating infectious disease of human and animals, caused by the organism *Mycobacterium tuberculosis* in humans and by *Mycobacterium bovis* in animals. The most common site of infection is the lungs, although other organs can be infected too.

Tularemia A bacterial disease of small animals, such as rabbits or rodents, which can be transmitted to humans by contact with biting insects such as flies, ticks, and mosquitoes. Thus, it is a "zoonoses." Symptoms include chills, fever, headache, joint pain, swollen lymph nodes, and even pneumonia if not treated by antibiotics.

Typhoid A severe bacterial infectious disease leading to massive dehydration due to diarrhea caused by ingestion of infected food or water. Other symptoms include high fever and a rose-colored rash. There is a vaccine to prevent typhoid.

Typhus A severe infectious disease caused by a small microorganism called rickettsia. It is spread through the bite of infected lice or fleas. Symptoms include high fever, rash, hacking cough, nausea, and vomiting.

Ulcers, gastric A perforated or small hole (also called a peptic ulcer) in the gastrointestinal tract, caused initially by the organism *Helicobacter pylori*. However, its ultimate cause is the destruction of the intestinal lining of the tract by hydrochloric acid and inflammatory factors overproduced by certain white blood cells attempting to destroy the microorganisms. Antibiotics are the most effective treatment.

Urease An enzyme that degrades urea to ammonia and water. It is an important enzyme produced by the pathogen that causes ulcers, *Helicobacter pylori*, because it renders the microenvironment where the organism thrives (the mucous of the intestinal lining) less acidic.

VacA toxin One of two toxins produced by *Helicobacter pylori* that destroy infected cells from within (known as a cytotoxin) and produce lesions characteristic of ulcers when injected into mice.

Vibrio cholerae The causative agent of cholera, a severe infectious disease of the small intestine that causes massive diarrhea, by consuming contaminated food or water.

Symptoms include cramps, excessive thirst, dryness of the skin, and nausea. The effects are due to the toxin produced by the microorganism. There is a vaccine to prevent the disease.

Virulence The comparative ability of a pathogen to cause disease. Also the characteristic factors that are produced by a pathogen.

Virus (virion) A submicroscopic entity consisting of one nucleic acid (DNA or RNA) surrounded by a protein coat, capable of being introduced into a living cell and of developing within that cell only. Separated into three general categories depending on their host: animal, plant, or bacterial.

Vitamin One of a number of organic compounds that exist in nature and function in very minute concentrations in living cells, aiding enzymes in carrying out their functions as biological catalysts.

White plague One of several names for tuberculosis, first used in the Middle Ages to describe some of the symptoms of the disease.

Wild type A genetic characterization of a microorganism that possesses no biochemical mutations when first isolated from nature.

Yeast A single-celled fungus that has lost its ability to grow in a filamentous (strand-like) form. Cultivated for its prodigious ability to ferment (catabolize) different substances to produce cheese and wine.

Yellow fever A deadly viral infection (usually fatal if not treated) spread by a bite from infected mosquitoes and causing hemorrhaging, whose symptoms include jaundice (or yellowing of the skin). There is no cure for yellow fever, but there is a preventative vaccine that is effective for many years.

Yersinia pestis The microorganism that causes bubonic plague, spread by the bite of an infected flea that was present on an infected rodent (usually a rat). One-quarter of the entire population of medieval Europe was wiped out by this plague.

Zoonoses Disease of animals that can be transmitted to humans (such as rabies).

PHOTO CREDITS

Chapter I.

1, 2, 3: ©Photo Researchers; 4: ©Cengage Learning; 5: ©George Eade; 6: ©Photo Researchers; 7: ©McGraw Hill, *Microbiology, a Human Perspective*, 4th ed. (New York, 2004); 8a, b, c, d: ©Cengage Learning.

Chapter II.

9, 10, 11, 12, 13, 14, 15, 16, 17, 18, 19, 20, 21: ©McGraw Hill, *Microbiology, a Human Perspective*, 4th ed. (New York, 2004).

Chapter III.

22: ©Granger Collection; 23a, 23b, 24, 25: ©Cengage Learning.

Chapter IV.

26: ©McGraw Hill, *Microbiology, a Human Perspective*, 5th ed. (New York, 2007); 27: ©Corbis; 28a, b: ©Phototake; 29: ©Photo Researches; 30: ©Corbis; 31: ©Phototake.

Chapter V.

32: ©Centers for Disease Control; 33a, 33b, 33c, 34, 35: ©McGraw Hill, *Microbiology, a Human Perspective*, 4th ed. (New York, 2004); 36: ©Custom Medical Stock Photo; 37: McGraw Hill, *Microbiology, a Human Perspective*, 4th ed. (New York, 2004); 38: ©Visuals Unlimited; 39: ©Peter Arnold; 40a, 40b, 41, 42: ©Benjamin Cummings, Brock, *Biology of Microorganisms*, 13th ed. (San Francisco, 2009); 43, 44: McGraw Hill, *Microbiology, a Human Perspective*, 4th ed. (New York, 2004).

Chapter VI.

45: ©Keith Kasnot.

Chapter VII.

46: ©Visuals Unlimited.

INDEX